CAMBRIDGE LIBRAR

Books of enduring sch

History of Medicine

It is sobering to realise that as recently as the year in which On the Origin of Species was published, learned opinion was that diseases such as typhus and cholera were spread by a 'miasma', and suggestions that doctors should wash their hands before examining patients were greeted with mockery by the profession. The Cambridge Library Collection reissues milestone publications in the history of Western medicine as well as studies of other medical traditions. Its coverage ranges from Galen on anatomical procedures to Florence Nightingale's common-sense advice to nurses, and includes early research into genetics and mental health, colonial reports on tropical diseases, documents on public health and military medicine, and publications on spa culture and medicinal plants.

An Account of the Nature and Medicinal Virtues of the Principal Mineral Waters of Great Britain and Ireland

Although he was tried for attempted murder and died in Newgate Prison, the natural philosopher and apothecary John Elliot (1747–87) published a number of significant scientific works in the first part of the 1780s, especially with regard to sensory perception. This 1789 second edition of a 1781 work is essentially an alphabetically arranged catalogue of the principal British mineral waters, their properties and uses, along with those 'most celebrated ones which the English valetudinarian may have occasion to visit on the continent'. In his introduction, Elliot classes the waters according to their respective mineral properties and supplies details of the four classes of substances found united with water, and three methods for analysis. An extract of Joseph Priestley's 1772 pamphlet *Directions for Impregnating Water with Fixed Air*, with Dr John Nooth's alternative method as an appendix, forms an entertaining preface, informative as to the history of producing carbonated water.

Cambridge University Press has long been a pioneer in the reissuing of out-of-print titles from its own backlist, producing digital reprints of books that are still sought after by scholars and students but could not be reprinted economically using traditional technology. The Cambridge Library Collection extends this activity to a wider range of books which are still of importance to researchers and professionals, either for the source material they contain, or as landmarks in the history of their academic discipline.

Drawing from the world-renowned collections in the Cambridge University Library and other partner libraries, and guided by the advice of experts in each subject area, Cambridge University Press is using state-of-the-art scanning machines in its own Printing House to capture the content of each book selected for inclusion. The files are processed to give a consistently clear, crisp image, and the books finished to the high quality standard for which the Press is recognised around the world. The latest print-on-demand technology ensures that the books will remain available indefinitely, and that orders for single or multiple copies can quickly be supplied.

The Cambridge Library Collection brings back to life books of enduring scholarly value (including out-of-copyright works originally issued by other publishers) across a wide range of disciplines in the humanities and social sciences and in science and technology.

An Account of the Nature and Medicinal Virtues of the Principal Mineral Waters of Great Britain and Ireland

And Those Most in Repute on the Continent

John Elliot

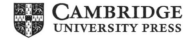

CAMBRIDGE
UNIVERSITY PRESS

University Printing House, Cambridge, CB2 8BS, United Kingdom

Published in the United States of America by Cambridge University Press, New York

Cambridge University Press is part of the University of Cambridge.
It furthers the University's mission by disseminating knowledge in the pursuit of
education, learning and research at the highest international levels of excellence.

www.cambridge.org
Information on this title: www.cambridge.org/9781108060165

© in this compilation Cambridge University Press 2013

This edition first published 1789
This digitally printed version 2013

ISBN 978-1-108-06016-5 Paperback

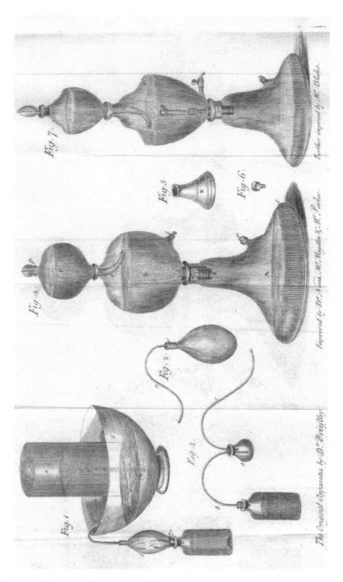

The material originally positioned here is too large for reproduction in this reissue. A PDF can be downloaded from the web address given on page iv of this book, by clicking on 'Resources Available'.

AN

ACCOUNT

OF THE

NATURE and MEDICINAL VIRTUES

OF THE

Principal Mineral Waters

OF

GREAT BRITAIN AND IRELAND;

AND THOSE

MOST IN REPUTE ON THE CONTINENT.

TO WHICH ARE PREFIXED

Directions for IMPREGNATING WATER with FIXED AIR, in order to communicate to it the peculiar Virtues of PYRMONT WATER, and other MINERAL WATERS of a similar Nature, extracted from Dr. PRIESTLEY's EXPERIMENTS ON AIR.

WITH AN APPENDIX,

Containing a Description of Dr. NOOTH's Apparatus, with the IMPROVEMENTS made in it by others. And a Method of IMPREGNATING WATER with HEPATIC AIR, so as to imitate the AIX-LA-CHAPELLE and other SULPHUREOUS WATERS.

By JOHN ELLIOT, M.D.

The Second Edition, corrected and enlarged.

LONDON:

PRINTED FOR J. JOHNSON, N°. 72, ST. PAUL'S CHURCH-YARD, MDCCLXXXIX.

ADVERTISEMENT
TO THE
FIRST EDITION.

DR. PRIESTLEY's Pamphlet on the Impregnation of Water with Fixed Air being out of print, and that Gentleman having no intention of republifhing it, I have judged proper to prefix it to the following Tract, with the additions, as printed in his fecond Volume of Experiments on Air. This was done as well that the reader might be entertained with the hiftory of the difcovery, as inftructed in an eafy method of making the impregnation when Dr. Nooth's apparatus might not be at hand.

J. E.

Newman Street,
Aug. 30, 1781.

IN this Second Edition the contents of the principal Waters, and their Proportions, when they could be obtained from any good authority, have been inferted: fome, which have come into repute fince the publication of the former edition, are added: the proportions of the ingredients for imitating different Mineral Waters have been altered, to bring them nearer to what, from the analyfes of later chemifts, we may prefume to be their true compofition: the method of preparing the mephitic alkaline water is given in a more full and improved manner; and that part which relates to the analyfis of waters is confiderably enlarged.

CONTENTS

OF THE IMPREGNATION OF WATER WITH
FIXED AIR.

AN ACCOUNT OF THE NATURE, PRO-
PERTIES, AND MEDICINAL VIR-
TUES OF THE PRINCIPAL MINE-
RAL WATERS IN GREAT BRITAIN
AND IRELAND.

OF THE

IMPREGNATION OF WATER

WITH

FIXED AIR.

From Dr. PRIESTLEY's Experiments, Vol. II.

CHAPTER I.

THE HISTORY OF THE DISCOVERY.

IT often amufes me when I review the hiftory of experimental philo-fophy, to obferve how very nearly one difcovery is connected with another, and yet that, for a long time, no per-fon fhall have perceived that con-nection, fo as to have been actually led from the one to the other; and efpecially that he who made the firft difcovery fhould ftop fhort in his pro-grefs, and not advance a fingle ftep

B   farther,

farther, to make the other, which was perhaps of infinitely more confequence. And yet the cafe may be fuch, that it fhall be fo far from requiring more genius, or ingenuity, to advance that other ftep, that it is rather a matter of wonder, how it was poffible for the moft common capacity to ftop fhort of it. We alfo frequently find that they who make the moft important philofophical difcoveries overlook the moft obvious *ufes* of them. Several ftriking examples of this kind wfll be found in my *Hiftory of electricity*, and alfo in the *Hiftory of difcoveries relating to vifion, light, and colours*.

In fuch cafes as thefe it behoves an hiftorian to be much on his guard, left he fhould haftily conclude that to have been fact which he only *imagines* muft have been fo, but for which no direct evidence can be produced. As this

✝   is

is a cafe of fome curiofity refpecting
the human mind, I fhall give an in-
ftance of it; and I am able to produce a very remarkable one relating
to the fubject of this fection.

When it was difcovered that the
acidulous tafte and peculiar virtues of
Pyrmont water, and other mineral
waters of a fimilar nature, were owing
to the fixed air which they contained;
when this air had been actually expelled from the water, and it was
found that the fame water, and even
other water, would reimbibe the fame
air; we are apt to conclude that the
perfon who made thefe difcoveries,
and efpecially the laft of them (who
alfo muft have known that fixed air
is a thing very eafy to be procured)
muft have immediately gone to work
to reduce this *theory* into *practice*, by
actually impregnating common water
with fixed air, in order to give it the

peculiar

peculiar virtues of thofe medicinal
mineral waters which are fo highly,
and fo juftly valued, and which are
procured at fo great an expence, efpecially in this country.   Accordingly, Dr. Nooth has advanced, Phil.
Tranf. vol. lxv. p. 59, that " the
" poffibility of impregnating water
" with fixed air was no fooner afcer-
" tained by experiment, than various
" methods were contrived to effect the
" impregnation;" and I doubt not
this ingenious philofopher impofed
upon himfelf in the manner defcribed
above. This, however, is fo far from
being the cafe, that I do not believe
it is poffible to produce the leaft evidence that any perfon had the thing
in view before the publication of my
pamphlet upon that fubject, in the
year 1772.

Indeed had this thing been fo much
as *an object of attention* to philofo-
phers,

phers, it is impoffible but that fome of them muft have hit upon a method that would have fufficiently fucceeded. Nay, the thing is fo very eafy, and the end attainable in fo many ways, that there muft have been, in a very fhort time, a great variety of methods to impregnate water with fixed air, as there are now; and we fhould cer-tainly have heard of *artificial mineral waters* being made according to them. It is impoffible not to conclude fo, when we confider the *time that has elapfed* fince the publication of all the difcoveries that led to it.

Dr. Brownrigg's paper, giving an account of his difcovery of fixed air in the Spa water, was read at the Royal Society June the 13th 1765, and was publifhed in 1766. This excellent philofopher compleatly de-compofed that mineral water, but he gives no hint of his having fo much

B 3   as

as attempted to *recompofe* it, or of
making a fimilar water, by impregnating common water with the fame
volatile principle. It is fufficiently
evident that he had not thought of
this, though we may wonder that he
fhould not have done it, becaufe he
has not mentioned it, as an object of
purfuit.

In the year following, Mr. Caven-
difh's valuable papers on the fubject
of factitious air were publifhed. He
firft afcertained how much fixed air
a given quantity of water could be
made to imbibe; yet it does not appear that he ever thought of *tafting*
the water, much lefs that he thought
of making any *practical ufe* of his difcovery.

If any negative argument can be
decifive, it is that in the year 1772,
the very year in which my pamphlet came out, Dr. Falconer publifhed
his

his excellent and elaborate treatife on
the *Bath waters,* in which he treats
very largely of mineral waters in general, and all their poffible impregnations ; and yet, though he treats of
fixed air as one ingredient in many of
them, fee p. 185, he drops no hint
about compofing fuch water, by im-
parting fixed air to common water.
Alfo on the 12th of September in the
fame year, Dr. Rutherford publifhed
his ingenious *Differtation on Fixed
Air,* in which he fpeaks of the prefence of it in Pyrmont water, p. 3,
but without giving the leaft hint of
his being acquainted with any method of imitating them. And yet,
Dr. Nooth fays, in fa&t, that from
the year 1766, at the lateft, *various
methods* were contrived to effe&t the
impregnation, though he allows that I
was the only perfon who " publifhed

" any defcription of an apparatus cal-
" culated entirely for this purpofe."

According to this account of the
matter there were, in the interval between 1766 and 1772, a fpace of fix
years, a variety of methods for impregnating water with fixed air, fome
of them prior to, and perhaps much
better than mine (though he gives no
hint of his own having been invented
in that period, but fpeaks of it as fug-
gefted by the confideration of the im-
perfection of mine) but that I happened to get the ftart in the publication. Dr. Falconer, however, though
the friend of Dr. Nooth (fee his treatife on Bath Water, vol. ii. p. 323)
had certainly never heard of any of
thofe methods, or even of mine, at
the very termination of that period;
and though my own acquaintance
with philofophical and medical people

ple is pretty extenfive, I never heard of any of the *various methods* that Dr. Nooth fpeaks of; nor fince the publication of my method have I heard of any perfon whatever having pretended to have done the fame thing before; though nothing is more common than fuch claims, and very often on the moft trifling pretences.

Mr. Venelle, indeed, immediately upon the tranflation of my pamphlet into French, which was within a few weeks after the publication of it in Englifh (owing to the laudable zeal of Mr. Trudaine, for promoting all philofophical and ufeful improvements) publifhed an extract of his papers from the *Memoires de Mathematique & de Phyfique*, to vindicate to himfelf not my difcovery, but, in fact, that of Dr. Brownrigg. However, what he pretends to have difcovered was, that the virtues of the acidulous wa-

ters

ters were owing to *air, in general,* without having any idea of the diffe-rence between fixed air and common air; fo that his difcovery was fo far from being the fame with mine, that it could not poffibly have led into it.

As I have hitherto only publifhed the method of impregnating water with fixed air in a fmall pamphlet, for the ufe of thofe who might chufe to reduce it into practice, without giv-ing any account of the manner in which the difcovery (if it deferves to be called one) was made, which has been my cuftom with refpect to every thing elfe, I fhall do it here; and I hope the narrative will not be altoge-ther difpleafing, as this bufinefs has gained fo much attention in all parts of Europe, as well as in England, and promifes in a fhort time to fave the very great expence of tranfporting acidulous

acidulous waters to confiderable dif-
tances, by fuperceding, in a great
meafure, the ufe of them. And
though what I have done in this bufinefs has certainly the leaft merit poffible with refpect to *ingenuity*, I fhall
always confider it as one of the *hap-
pieft* thoughts that ever occurred to
me; becaufe it has proved to be of
very fignal *benefit* to mankind, and
will, I doubt not, be of much more
confequence in a courfe of time.

It was a little after Midfummer in
1767, that I removed from Warring-
ton to Leeds; and living, for the firft
year, in a houfe that was contiguous
to a large common brewery, fo good
an opportunity produced in me an inclination to make fome experiments
on the fixed air that was conftantly
produced in it. Had it not been for
this circumftance, I fhould, probably,
never have attended to the fubject of

air

air at all. Happening to have read
Dr. Brownrigg's excellent paper on
the Spa water about the fame time,
one of the firft things that I did in
this brewery was to place fhallow
veffels of water within the region of
fixed air, on the furface of the fermenting veffels; and having left them all
night, I generally found, the next
morning, that the water had acquired
a very fenfible and pleafant impregnation; and it was with peculiar fa-
tisfaction that I firft drank of this
water, which I believe was the firft
of its kind that had ever been tafted
by man.

This procefs, however, was very
flow. But after fome time it occurred to me, that the impregnation
might be accelerated, by pouring the
water from one veffel into another,
while they were both held within the
fphere of the fixed air; and accordingly

ingly I found that I could do as much in about five minutes in this way, as I had been able to do in many hours before. Several of my friends who vifited me while I lived in that houfe will remember my taking them into that brewery, and giving them a glafs of this artificial Pyrmont water, made in their prefence. Among others, I will take the liberty to mention John Lee, Efq; of Lincoln's Inn, who was particularly ftruck with the contrivance, and the effect of it. This was in the fummer of the year 1768.

One would naturally think, that having actually impregnated common water with fixed air, produced in a brewery, I fhould immediately have fet about doing the fame thing with air fet loofe from chalk, &c. by fome of the ftronger acids; and I do remember that it did occur to me that the thing was poffible. But, eafy as

the

the practice proved to be, no method
of doing it at that time occurred to
me. I ſtill continued to make my
Pyrmont water in the manner above
mentioned 'till I left that ſituation,
which was about the end of the ſummer 1768 ; and from that time, being
engaged in other ſimilar purſuits, with
the reſult of which the public are acquainted, I made no more of the Pyrmont water 'till the ſpring of the
year 1772.

In the mean time I had acquainted
all my friends with what I had done,
and frequently expreſſed my wiſhes
that perſons who had the care of
large *diſtilleries* (where I was told that
fermentation was much ſtronger than
in common breweries) would contrive
to have veſſels of water ſuſpended
within the fixed air, which they produced, with a farther contrivance for
agitating the ſurface of the water ; as
I did

I did not doubt but that, by this means, they might, with little or no expence, make great quantities of Pyrmont water; by which they might at the fame time both ferve the Public, and benefit themfelves. For I never had the moft diftant thought of making any advantage of the fcheme myfelf.

In all this time, viz. from 1767 to 1772, I never heard of any method of impregnating water with fixed air but that above mentioned. My thinking at all of reducing to practice any method of effecting this, by air diflodged from chalk, and other calcareous fubftances, was owing to a mere accident. Being at dinner with the Duke of Northumberland, in the fpring of the year laft mentioned, his Grace produced a bottle of water diftilled by Dr. Irving for the ufe of the navy. This water was perfectly fweet, but, like

like all diftilled water, wanted the
brifknefs and fpirit of frefh fpring water; when it immediately occurred to
me that I could eafily mend that water for the ufe of the navy, and perhaps fupply them with an eafy and
cheap method of preventing or curing
the fea-fcurvy, viz. by impregnating
it with fixed air. For having been
bufy about a year before with my experiments on air, in the courfe of
which I had afcertained the propor-
tional quantity of feveral kinds of air
that given quantities of water would
take up, I was at no lofs for the *method* of doing it in general, viz. in-
verting a jar filled with water, and
conveying air into it from bladders
previoufly filled with air.   This
fcheme I immediately mentioned to
the Duke and the company, who all
feemed to be much pleafed with it,
and expreffed their wifhes that I would
attend

attend to it, and endeavour to reduce it into practice; which I promised to do.

The next day I provided a small apparatus, adapted to this purpose, at my lodgings, which was very easy, as it required no other veffels but such as are in constant family use, and with this I presently impregnated a quantity of the New River water, so as to make it imbibe about its bulk of air. But I was far from having hit upon the *easiest method* of doing it; for my jars were of an equal width throughout. However, with these veffels the process was compleated in about twenty minutes, or half an hour.

A few days after this, having an invitation to wait upon Sir George Savile, I carried with me a bottle of my impregnated water, and told him the use that might be made of it, viz. that of supplying a pleasant and whole-

fome

fome beverage for feamen, and fuch as might probably prevent or cure the fea-fcurvy. Sir George, with that warmth with which he efpoufes every thing that he conceives to be for the public good, infifted upon writing a card immediately to Lord Sandwich, propofing to introduce me to him, as having *a propofal for the ufe of the navy.* As I could make no objection, the card was accordingly written, and an anfwer was prefently returned from his Lordfhip, informing us that he would be glad to fee us the next day. Upon this I drew up fomething in the form of a *propofal,* which, accompanied by Sir George, I prefented to his Lordfhip, who promifed to lay it before the Board of Admiralty.

Prefently after this I had notice from the Secretary to the Board of Admiralty, that the *College of Phyfi-cians* were appointed to examine my propofal,

propofal, and to make their report of it to the Board, and an early day was fixed for me to wait upon them at their hall in Warwick-Lane; where, before a very full meeting, I produced a bottle of my impregnated water, and alfo, at their requeft, fetched my apparatus, and fhewed them the manner in which I had impregnated it. There were prefent feveral of the moft eminent phyficians in London; but both the *fcheme* and the *objeɛƚ* of it, appeared to be entirely new to every one of them; and moft of them feemed to be much pleafed with it.

Accordingly, a favourable report was made to the Board of Admiralty, and I was acquainted by the Secretary, that the Captains of the two fhips which were juft then failing for the South-Seas had orders to make a trial of the impregnated water; and for their ufe I drew out my *Direɛƚions*
in

in writing, and fent a drawing of
the neceffary apparatus. The method
which I had now got into was a great
improvement upon that which I had
made ufe of before the College of
Phyficians. For, in confequence of
giving more attention to it, I had, by
that time, brought it to the ftate in
which it is defcribed in the pamphlet.

In the mean time, I had, before I
left London, in the fpring of that year,
made the experiment of the impregnation of water with fixed air in the
prefence of moft of my philofophical
acquaintance, and their friends, both
at my own lodgings, and in other
places. But upon none of thefe occafions did it appear that any of them
had heard of any other perfon having
had the fame thing in view.

Laftly, I will obferve, that Sir John
Pringle, in his *Difcourfe on different
kinds*

kinds of air (in which he has, with the greateſt exactneſs, aſſigned to every perſon concerned in theſe diſcoveries their due ſhare of praiſe) gives no hint of his being acquainted with any other method of impregnating water with fixed air, than that which I had publiſhed. He certainly had not heard of any of thoſe to which Dr. Nooth alludes.

As I have not to this day, directly or indirectly, made the leaſt advantage of this ſcheme; but, on the contrary, am juſt ſo much a loſer by it as the experiments coſt me, I think it is not too much for the Public to allow me, what I believe is ſtrictly my due, *the ſole merit of the diſcovery*; which with reſpect to *ingenuity*, or ſagacity, is next to nothing; but with reſpect to its *utility* is, unqueſtionably, of un-ſpeakable value to my country and to mankind.

CHAP-

CHAPTER II.

DIRECTIONS FOR IMPREGNATING WATER WITH FIXED AIR.

Sect. 1. *The Preface to the Directions as first published.*

THE method of impregnating water with fixed air, of which a de-scription is given in this pamphlet, I hit upon in a course of experiments; an account of which was lately communicated to the Royal Society; containing observations on several different kinds of air, with only a hint of the method of combining this parti-cular kind with water or other fluids. Judging that water thus impregnated with fixed air must be particularly fer-viceable in long voyages, by prevent-ing or curing the sea-scurvy, accord-ing to the theory of Dr. Macbride;

and

and all the Phyficians of my acquaintance concurring with me in that opinion, I made the firft communication of it to the Lords of the Admiralty, who referred me to the College of Phyficians; and thofe gentlemen being pleafed to make a report favourable to the fcheme, a trial has been ordered to be made of it on board fome of his Majefty's fhips. To make this procefs more generally known, and that more frequent trials may be made by water thus medicated, at land as well as at fea, I have been induced to make the prefent publication.

Sir John Pringle firft obferved, that putrefaction was checked by fermentation; and Dr. Macbride difcovered that this effect was produced by the fixed air which is generated in that procefs, and upon that principle recommended the ufe of *wort*, as fupplying a quantity of this fixed air, by fermen-

fermentation in the ftomach, in the
fame manner as it is done by frefh
vegetables, for which he, therefore,
thought that it would be a fubftitute;
and experience has confirmed his
conjecture.   Dr. Black found that
lime - ftone, and all calcareous fubftances, contain fixed air, that the prefence of it makes them what is called
mild, and that the eprivation of it
renders them *cauftic*; Dr. Brownrigg
farther difcovered that Pyrmont, and
other mineral waters, which have the
fame acidulous tafte, contain a confiderable proportion of this very kind
of air, and that upon this their peculiar fpirit and virtues depend; and I
think myfelf fortunate in having hit
upon a very eafy method of communicating this air to any kind of water,
or, indeed, to almoft any fluid fubftance.   In fhort, by this method this
great antifeptic principle may be ad-
ministered

miniftered in a great variety of agreeable vehicles.

If this difcovery (though it doth
not deferve that name) be of any ufe
to my countrymen, and to mankind
at large, I fhall have my reward. For
this purpofe I have made the communication as early as I conveniently
could, fince the lateft improvements
that I have made in the procefs ; and
I cannot help exprefling my wifhes,
that all perfons, who difcover any
thing that promifes to be generally
ufeful, would adopt the fame method.

Sect. 2.   *The Directions.*

If water be only in contact with
fixed air, it will begin to imbibe it,
but the mixture is greatly accelerated
by agitation, which is continually
bringing frefh particles of air and water into contact.   All that is neceffary, therefore, to make this procefs

C   expeditious

expeditious and effectual, is firft to
procure a fufficient quantity of this
fixed air, and then to contrive a method by which the air and water may
be ftrongly agitated in the fame veffel,
without any danger of admitting the
common air to them; and this is eafily done by firft filling any veffel with
water, and introducing the fixed air
to it, while it ftands inverted in another veffel of water. That every
part of the procefs may be as intelli-
gible as poffible, even to thofe who
have no previous knowledge of the
fubject, I fhall defcribe it very mi-
nutely, fubjoining feveral remarks and
obfervations relating to varieties in the
procefs, and other things of a mif-
cellaneous nature.

The Preparation.

Take a glafs veffel, *a*, fig. 1.
with a pretty narrow neck, but fo
formed,

formed, that it will ftand upright with its mouth downwards, and having filled it with water, lay a flip of clean paper, or thin pafteboard, upon it. Then, if they be preffed clofe together, the veffel may be turned up- fide down, without danger of admit- ting common air into it; and when it is thus inverted, it muft be placed in another yeffel, in the form of a bowl or bafon, *b*, with a little water in it, fo much as to permit the flip of paper or pafteboard to be withdrawn, and the end of the pipe *c* to be in- troduced.

This pipe muft be flexible, and air- tight, for which purpofe it is, I be- lieve, beft made of leather, fewed with a waxed thread, in the manner ufed by fhoe-makers. Into both ends of this pipe a piece of a quill fhould be thruft, to keep them open, while one of them is introduced into the

veffel of water, and the other into the
bladder *d*, the oppofite end of which
is tied round a cork, which muft be
perforated, the hole being kept open
by a quill; and the cork muft fit a
phial *e*, two thirds of which fhould
be filled with chalk juft covered with
water.

I have fince, however, found it moft
convenient to ufe a *glafs tube*, and to
preferve the advantage which I had,
of agitating the veffel *e*, I have *two
bladders*, communicating by a perforated cork, to which they are both
tied.   For one bladder would hardly
give room enough for that purpofe.

The Procefs.

Things being thus prepared, and
the phial containing the chalk and
water being detached from the bladder,
and the pipe alfo from the veffel of
water, pour a little oil of vitriol upon
the

the chalk and water; and having carefully preffed all the common air out of the bladder, put the cork into the bottle prefently after the effervef- cence has begun. Alfo prefs the blad- der once more after a little of the newly generated air has got into it, in order the more effectually to clear it of all the remains of the common air; and then introduce the end of the pipe into the mouth of the veffel of water as in the drawing, and begin to agitate the chalk and water brifkly. This will prefently produce a confiderable quantity of fixed air, which will dif- tend the bladder; and this being preffed, the air will force its way through the pipe, and afcend into the veffel of water, the water at the fame time defcending, and coming into the bafon.

When about one half of the water is forced out, let the operator lay his

hand

hand upon the uppermoſt part of the
veſſel, and ſhake it as briſkly as he
can, not to throw the water out of
the baſon ; and in a few minutes the
water will abſorb the air ; and taking
its place, will nearly fill the veſſel as
at the firſt.   Then ſhake the phial
containing the chalk and water again,
and force more air into the veſſel, 'till,
upon the whole, about an equal bulk
of air has been thrown into it.   Alſo
ſhake the water as before, 'till no
more of the air can be imbibed.   As
ſoon as this is perceived to be the
eaſe, the water is ready for uſe ; and
if it be not uſed immediately, ſhould
be put into a bottle as ſoon as poſſi-
ble, well corked, and cemented.   It
will keep, however, very well, if the
bottle be only well corked, and kept
with the mouth downwards.

Obſerva-

Obſervations.

1. The baſon may be placed inverted upon the veſſel full of water, with a ſlip of paper between them, and then both turned upſide down together; but all this trouble will be ſaved by having a larger veſſel of water, in which both of them may be immerſed.

2. If the veſſel containing the water to be agitated be large, it may be moſt convenient firſt to place it inverted, in a baſon full of water, and then to draw out the common air by means of a ſyphon, either making uſe of a ſyringe, or drawing it out with the mouth. In' this caſe, alſo, ſome kind of handle ſhould be faſtened to the bottom of the veſſel, for the more eaſy agitation of it.

3. A narrow-mouthed veſſel is not neceſſary, but it is the moſt proper for

the

the purpofe, becaufe it may be agitated with lefs danger of the common air getting into it.

4. The flexible pipe is not necef-fary, though I think it is exceedingly convenient. When it is not ufed, a bent tube, *a*, fig. 2. (for which glafs is the moft proper) muft be ready to be inferted into the hole made in the cork, when the bladder containing the fixed air is feparated from the phial, in which it was generated. The extremity of this tube being put un-der the veffel of water, and the blad-der being compreffed, the air will be conveyed into it, as before.

5. If the ufe of a bladder be ob-jected to, though nothing can be more inoffenfive, the phial containing the chalk and water muft not be agitated at all, or with the greateft caution; unlefs a fmall phial, *a*, fig. 3. be in-terpofed between the phial and the

veffel

veffel of water, in the manner repre-
fented in the drawing. For by this
means the chalk and water that may
be thrown up the tube *b* will lodge at
the bottom of the phial *a*, while nothing but the air will get into the
pipe *c*, and fo enter the water. If the
tube *b* be made of tin or copper, the
fmall phial *a* will not need any other
fupport, the cork into which the ex-
tremities of both the tubes are inferted being made to fit the phial very
exactly.

6. The phial *e*, fig. 1. fhould always be placed, or held, confiderably
lower than the veffel *a* ; that if any
part of the mixture fhould be thrown
up into the bladder, it may remain in
the lower part of it, from which it
may be eafily preffed back again.
This, however, is not neceffary, fince
if it remain in the lower part of the
bladder, nothing but the pure air will

C 5   get

get into the pipe, and fo into the water.

7. If much more than half of the veffel be filled with air, there will not be a body of water fufficient to agitate, and the procefs will take up much more time.

8. If the chalk be too finely powdered, it will yield the fixed air too faft.

9. After every procefs, the water to which the chalk is put muft be changed.

10. It will be proper to fill the bladder with water once every day, after it has been ufed, that any of the oil of vitriol which may have got into it, and would be in danger of corroding it, may be thoroughly diluted.

11. The veffel, which I have generally made ufe of, holds about three pints, and the phial containing the chalk and water is one of ten ounces; and

and I find that a little more than a tea-fpoonful of oil of vitriol is fufficient to produce as much air as will impregnate that quantity of water.

12. If the veffel containing the water be larger, the phial containing the chalk and the oil of vitriol fhould either be larger in proportion, or frefh water and oil of vitriol muft be put to the chalk, to produce the requifite quantity of air.

13. In general, the whole procefs does not take up more than about a quarter of an hour, the agitation not five minutes; and in nearly the fame time might a veffel of water, containing two or three gallons, or indeed any quantity that a perfon could well fhake, be impregnated with fixed air, if the phial containing the chalk and oil of vitriol, be larger in the fame proportion.

14. To give the water as much air

C 6 as

as it can receive in this way, the procefs may be repeated with the water
thus impregnated. I generally chufe
to do it two or three times, but very
little will be gained by repeating it of-
tener; fince, after fome time, as much
fixed air will efcape from that part of
the furface of the water which is expofed to the common air, as can be
imbibed from within the veffel.

15. All calcareous fubftances contain fixed air, and any acids may be
ufed in order to fet it loofe from
them; but chalk and oil of vitriol
are, both of them, the cheapeft, and,
upon the whole, the beft for the purpofe.

16. It may poffibly be imagined
that part of the oil of vitriol is rendered volatile in this procefs, and fo
becomes mixed with the water; but
it does not appear, by the moft rigid
chymical examination, that the leaft
perceivable

perceivable quantity of the acid gets into the water in this way; and if fo fmall a quantity as a fingle drop of oil of vitriol be mixed with a pint of water (and a much greater quantity would be far from making it lefs wholefome) it might be difcovered. The experiments which were made to afcertain this fact were made with *diftilled water*, the difagreeable tafte of which is not taken off, in any degree, by the mixture of fixed air. Other-wife, diftilled water, being clogged with no foreign principle, will imbibe fixed air fafter, and retain a greater quantity of it than other water. In the experiments that were made for this purpofe, I was affifted by Mr. Hey, a furgeon in Leeds, who is well fkilled in the methods of examining the properties of mineral waters.

17. Dr. Brownrigg, who made his experiments on Pyrmont water at the fpring

fpring head, never found that it contained fo much as one half of an eqùal
bulk of air; but in this method the
water is eafily made to imbibe an
equal bulk. For it muft be obferved,
that a confiderable quantity of the
moft foluble part of the air is incor-
porated with the water, as it firft
afcends through it, before it occupies
its place in the upper part of the
veffel.

18. The heat of boiling water will
expel all the fixed air, if a phial containing this impregnated water be held
in it; but it will often require above
half an hour to effect it compleatly.

19. If any perfon would chufe to
make this medicated water more nearly
to refemble genuine Pyrmont water,
Sir John Pringle informs me, that
from eight to ten drops of *Tinctura
Martis cum fpiritu falis* muft be mixed
with every pint of it. It is agreed,
however,

however, on all hands, that the peculiar virtues of Pyrmont, or any other mineral water which has the fame brifk or acidulous tafte, depend not upon its being a chalybeate, but upon the fixed air which it contains.

But water impregnated with fixed air does of itfelf diffolve iron, as the ingenious Mr. Lane has difcovered; and iron filings put to this medicated water make a ftrong and agreeable chalybeate, fimilar to fome other natural chalybeates, which hold the iron in folution by means of fixed air only, and not by means of any acid; and thefe chalybeates, I am informed, are generally the moft agreeable to the ftomach.

20. By this procefs may fixed air be given to wine, beer, and almoft any liquor whatever : and when beer is become flat or dead, it will be revived by this means; but the delicate agreeable

able flavour, or acidulous tafte communicated by the fixed air, and which is manifeft in water, will hardly be perceived in wine, or other liquors which have much tafte of their own.

21. I would not interfere with the province of the phyfician, but I cannot entirely fatisfy myfelf without taking this opportunity to fuggeft fuch hints as have occurred to myfelf, or my friends, with refpect to the *medicinal ufes* of water impregnated with fixed air, and alfo of fixed air in other applications.

In general, the difeafes in which water impregnated with fixed air will moft probably be ferviceable, are thofe of a *putrid* nature, of which kind is the *fea-fcurvy*. It can hardly be doubted, alfo, but that this water muft have all the medicinal virtues of Pyrmont water, and of other mineral waters fimilar to it, whatever they be; efpecially especially if a few iron filings be put to it, to render it a chalybeate, like genuine Pyrmont water. It is possible, however, that in some cases it may be desirable to have the *fixed air* of Pyrmont water, without the *iron* which it contains.

Having this opportunity, I shall also hint the application of fixed air in the form of *clysters,* which occurred to me while I was attending to this subject, as what promises to be useful to correct putrefaction in the inteftinal canal, and other parts of the fystem to which it may, by this channel, be conveyed. It has been tried once by Mr. Hey above-mentioned, and the recovery of the patient from an alarming putrid fever, when the stools were become black, hot, and very fetid, was so circumstanced, that it is not improbable but that it might be owing, in some measure, to those clysters.

clyfters.   The application, however,
appeared to be perfectly eafy and
fafe.

I cannot help thinking that fixed
air might be applied externally to
good advantage in other cafes of a putrid nature, even when the whole fyftem was affected. There would be
no difficulty in placing the body fo,
that the greateft part of its furface
fhould be expofed to this kind of air;
and if a piece of putrid flefh will become firm and fweet in that fituation,
as Dr. Macbride found, fome advantage, I fhould think, might be ex-
pected from the fame antifeptic application, affifted by the *vis vitæ*, operating internally, to counteract the
fame putrid tendency. Some Indians,
I have been informed, bury their patients, labouring under putrid difeafes, up to the chin in frefh mould,
which is alfo known to take off the
foetor

fœtor from flefh meat beginning to putrify. If this practice be of any ufe, may it not be owing to the fixed air imbibed by the pores of the fkin in that fituation? Following the plough is an old prefcription for a confumption, as alfo is living near lime kilns. There is often fome good reafon for very old and long continued practices, though it is frequently a long time before it be difcovered, and the *rationale* of them fatisfactorily explained.

Being no phyfician, I run no rifque by throwing out thefe random hints and conjectures. I fhall think myfelf happy, if any of them fhould be the means of making thofe perfons, whom they immediately concern, attend more particularly to the fubject. My friend Dr. Percival has for fome time paft been employed in making experiments on fixed air, and he is particularly attentive

tentive to the medicinal ufes of it;
and from his knowledge as a philofopher, and fkill in his profeffion, I
have very confiderable expectations.

CHAP-

CHAPTER III.

OF DR. NOOTH'S OBJECTIONS TO
THE PRECEDING METHOD OF
IMPREGNATING WATER WITH
FIXED AIR, AND A COMPARISON
OF IT WITH HIS OWN METHOD,
BOTH AS PUBLISHED BY HIM-
SELF, AND AS IMPROVED BY
MR. PARKER.

I can eafily forgive Dr. Nooth for his reprefenting me as having no other merit than the *firſt publication* of the method for impregnating water with fixed air, accounting for it as I have done before; but I cannot fo eafily forgive another paragraph in his paper, the tendency of which is intirely to difcredit a method, which, though it is, in fome refpects, inferior to his own, has neverthelefs its peculiar advantages:

vantages : and every advantage cannot poffibly concur in any one method. He fays, p. 59, " Independent
" of the inconveniencies attending
" the procefs, there was another ob-
" jection to the apparatus, which,
" with moft people, might have
" confiderable weight. The *bladder,*
" which formed part of it, was
" thought to render the water offen-
" five ; and when the folvent power
" of fixed air is confidered, it will not
" appear improbable, that the water
" would be always more or lefs taint-
" ed by the bladder. In fome trials
" which I made with Dr. Prieftley's
" apparatus, it always happened that
" the water acquired an *urinous fla-*
" *vour* ; and this tafte was, in gene-
" ral, fo predominant, that it could
" not be fwallowed without fome de-
" gree of reluctance."

That Dr. Nooth *did* produce an
impregnated

impregnated water which he could not fwallow without reluctance, and even that, in the trials to which he refers, he *generally* produced fuch water, I am far from doubting; becaufe that might happen from various caufes. But that the urinous flavour came from the *bladder*, as fuch, I will venture to fay is not poffible. For then it would *always* have had the fame effect; and not only myfelf have never perceived fuch a flavour as the Doctor complains of, but this is the only complaint of the kind that I have hitherto heard of; though many perfons of the moft delicate tafte, and particularly many ladies, have ufed the water impregnated in my method for months together. Few perfons have had to do with bladders, and fixed air confined in bladders, more than myfelf; and yet I have never feen any reafon to fufpect this great

folvent

folvent power of fixed air with refpect
to them ; efpecially fo as to be appa-
rent in the fpace of a few minutes.

But fuppofing the fixed air to be
capable of diffolving the whole bladder, and to carry it along with itfelf
into the impregnated water, no phyfician, or philofopher, will pretend to
fay that it could have any more tendency to give it an *urinous flavour*,
than if it had been any other mem-
brane of the animal body.

Indeed, as the Doctor himfelf does
not pretend to fay that this ftrange
urinous flavour was the effect of *all*
the impregnations of water made in
my method, but only in *fome* of them
(though it was *generally* fo, in thofe
particular trials) it is evident, from
his tacit confeffion, that it muft have
been an *accidental thing*, and could not
have come from the bladder, which I
fuppofe he made ufe of in all trials.

For

For he has not done me the juftice to acknowledge that, in my pamphlet, among the various methods of effecting the impregnation of water, I have defcribed one in which no bladder is made ufe of. When the Doctor fhall once more produce this urinous flavour (and as a new and curious experiment, it is certainly worthy of his farther inveftigation) taking care that no carelefs fervant fhall have mixed any urine in the water that he calls for, I fhall give this new objection to my procefs a farther examination. At prefent I am inclined to confider this as an experiment of the fervant, rather than of the Doctor himfelf.

Several perfons have thought that fixed air difcharged from *impure chalk* gives the water that is impregnated with it a dilagreeable flavour, but this I have never obferved myfelf; and any other calcareous matter may be

D ufed

uſed in my method, as well as in
that of Dr. Nooth, who recommends
chalk, as the beſt upon the whole.

I ſhall conclude theſe animadver-
ſions with doing what Dr. Nooth ought
to have done before me, viz. fairly
ſtating the advantages and diſadvan-
tages of our two methods.   His method requires *leſs ſkill* in the operator
and *a leſs conſtant attention*.   It is alſo
more elegant and cleanly, I mean with
reſpect to the *operator*; for this does
not at all affect the *impregnated water*.
On theſe accounts I generally recom-
mend and make uſe of his method
myſelf, eſpecially as the glaſſes are
made with improvements by Mr.
Parker.   But if Dr. Nooth be can-
did, he muſt acknowledge that my
method requires much *leſs time*, and
is much *leſs expenſive*; and therefore
muſt be more proper when a great
quantity of impregnated water is wanted;

ed.; and efpecially when there is but little room to make it in.

My method indeed requires a conftant attendance, but I queftion whether, upon the whole, more than is neceffary to be given to Dr. Nooth's method at intervals, if the water be at all agitated; confidering that mine does not require one-tenth part of the time. And though my method requires fome little fkill and addrefs, it is not fo much, but that many perfons, altogether unufed to experiments, have, to my knowledge, fucceeded in it very well, and have made the impregnated water in a conftant way for their family ufe, and without any affiftance befides what they got from the printed directions. My apparatus cofts little or nothing, becaufe no veffels are made for the purpofe; and both the chalk and the acids are made to go as far as poffible, by means

of

of the convenient agitation of the veffel in which they are contained. Whereas Dr. Nooth's method requires a peculiar and expenfive apparatus, and more wafte is unavoidable in the ufe of it. However, for the reafons abovementioned, I have never recommended my own method for the ufe of a family fince I have been acquainted with his.

What I have faid above is rather applicable to the apparatus as it is made by Mr. Parker, than to that which Dr. Nooth has defcribed. For Mr. Parker's glaffes are, in my opinion, confiderably improved from thofe of Dr. Nooth. It may be faid that the improvements confift in *little things*; but little things may have great effects; and, after the difcovery of the *firft method* of accomplifhing this end, all *fubfequent methods* may be called little things; and they may be end-
lefsly

lefsly diverfified, without any great claim of merit. I have feen feveral very ingenious methods fince the publication of mine, though none that I liked fo much, upon the whole, as that of Dr. Nooth, improved by Mr. Parker.

In Dr. Nooth's apparatus, if any more air than is wanted be produced, the water will run out of the uppermoft veffel. To ufe his own words, p. 63, " Should more air be extricat-
" ed than is fufficient, in the conduct
" of the procefs, to fill that veffel,
" the water will run over the top of
" it, and will continue to run as long
" as any air afcends in the middle vef-
" fel, or 'till the furface of the water
" is below the extremity of the bent
" tube; and in this cafe the whole
" would be wet and difagreeable."
But this difagreeable confequence can never happen in the ufe of Mr. Par-

ker's

ker's glaffes, becaufe the bent tube in
which the uppermoft veffel terminates is made of fuch a length, that
the water expelled from the middle
veffel can do no more than nearly fill
the uppermoft, and can never run
over; fo that whereas Dr. Nooth's
apparatus requires a conftant attendance, Mr. Parker's requires none.
The materials being once put into it,
the procefs will go on of itfelf, without any farther care; unlefs the operator fhould chufe to accelerate the
impregnation by now and then letting
out the air that is not eafily abforbed,
and by agitating the water. This I
think to be a confiderable advantage
gained by a very eafy contrivance of
Mr. Parker's, overlooked by Dr.
Nooth.

Mr. Parker derives another confiderable advantage from a *channel*
which he cuts in the ftopper of his
upper-

uppermoft veffel, or from a ftopper with a hole through the middle, which Dr. Nooth has not in his ; fo that either the operator muft be careful to take it out during the effervefcence, or it will be driven out, or fome of the veffels will burft, to the great danger of the by-ftanders; which actually happened in one made by Mr. Parker, before he thought of this method to prevent it. Whereas, through the channel in Mr. Parker's apparatus, the common air eafily efcapes from the uppermoft veffel, to make room for the water to afcend; and when, in the continuance of the procefs, the fixed air rifes through the bent tube into the uppermoft veffel, it lodges upon the furface of the water in it; and the communication between it and the common air being fo much obftructed, they are fufficiently feparated; fo that even the wa-

ter

ter in the uppermoſt veſſel has (if the
production of air be copious) almoſt
as much advantage for receiving the
impregnation, as that in the middle
veſſel.   This advantage Dr. Nooth
loſes.

Alſo, when he chuſes to ſeparate
the two uppermoſt veſſels from the
loweſt, in order to agitate the water,
he muſt either leave the mouth of the
uppermoſt veſſel open, in which caſe
he can hardly agitate the water at all;
or (as he prefers to do it) he muſt
put the ſtopper in, and conſequently
admit the common air to paſs his
valve, and mix with the fixed air,
which muſt greatly retard the abſorp-
tion of it: whereas Mr. Parker's veſſels may be agitated with the ſtopper
in, which, admitting the common air
into the upper veſſel, through the
channel cut in it (or through the hole
of the ſtopper) permits the water to
defcend

1

defcend into the lower, on the furface
of which nothing but fixed air is in-
cumbent. Should any common air
enter by the valve, which in this cafe
it hardly would, the finger of the perfon who fhakes the veffel may eafily
be placed fo as to prevent it.

Laftly, I confider it as a valuable
improvement in Mr. Parker's apparatus, that, by means of the openings
into the middle and loweft veffels,
clofed with ground ftopples, the operator is enabled to draw off his water, in order to tafte it occafionally,
or to add to his oil of vitriol or chalk,
&c. at pleafure, without giving himfelf the trouble of feparating the veffels
fels from one another for thofe purpofes.

The firft apparatus that I faw of
Mr. Parker's had no *valve* at all, but
only a glafs ftopple, with one or more
fmall perforations, for the afcent of

the

the air into the middle veſſel. This
I ſtill generally make uſe of, without
finding any occaſion for a valve; the
aſcent of the fixed air ſufficiently preventing the deſcent of the water, as
long as the proceſs continues, eſpecially when pounded *marble* is uſed.
This ſubſtance Dr. Franklin recommended to me, and I give it the pre-
ference very greatly to chalk, chiefly
on account of the length of time that
is required to expel the air from it:
For without any freſh acid, it will
often continue to yield air for ſeveral
days together.

That thoſe perſons who are not
poſſeſſed of the Engliſh *Philoſophical
Tranſactions*, and particularly foreign-
ers, may underſtand what has preceded, I ſhall give a drawing of Dr.
Nooth's apparatus *, as improved by

* Fig. 4.

Mr.

Mr. Parker, with the following general defcription of it.

In the loweft veffel, the chalk or marble, and the water acidulated with oil of vitriol, muft be put, and into the middle veffel the water to be impregnated. During the effervefcence, the fixed air rifes into the middle veffel, and refts upon the furface of the water in it, while the water that is difplaced by the air rifes through the bent tube into the uppermoft veffel, the common air going out through the channel in the ftopple. When the bent tube is of a proper length, the procefs requires no attention; and if the production of air be copious, the water will generally be fufficiently impregnated in five or fix hours. At leaft, all the attention that needs be given to it is to raife the uppermoft veffel once or twice, to let out that part of the fixed air which is not

readily

readily abforbed by water. If the operator chufe to accelerate the pro-cefs, by agitating the water, he muft feparate the two uppermoft veffels from the loweft. For if he fhould agitate them all together, he will oc-cafion too copious a production of air; and he will alfo be in danger of throwing the liquor contained in the loweft veffel into contact with the ftopple which feparates it from the middle veffel, by which means fome of the oil of vitriol might get into the water.

End of the Extract from Dr. PRIEST-LEY'S *Experiments on Air,* Vol. II.

APPEN-

APPENDIX.

DR. NOOTH'S METHOD OF IMPREG-
NATING WATER WITH FIXED
AIR, AS IMPROVED BY MR. PAR-
KER, MR. MAGELLAN, &c.

Defcription of the Apparatus.

See Fig. 4.

IT is made of glafs, and ftands on a
wooden veffel *d d* refembling a
tea-board, to catch any water that
may chance to be fpilled, and prevent
it from falling on the table. The
middle veffel B has a neck which is
inferted into the mouth of the veffel
A, to which it is ground air-tight.
This lower neck of the veffel B, has a
glafs ftopple S, compofed of two
parts, both having holes fufficient to

let

let a good quantity of air pafs through
them. Between thefe two parts
(which may be confidered as two
ftopples) is left a fmall fpace, containing a plano convex lens, (that is,
a glafs round on one fide and flat on
the other) which acts like a valve, in
letting the air pafs from below upwards, and hindering its return into
the veffel A.

The upper veffel C terminates below in a tube *r t,* which being crooked, hinders the immediate afcent of
the bubbles of fixed air into that veffel, before they reach the furface of the
water in the veffel B. The veffel C
is alfo ground air-tight to the upper
neck of the middle veffel B, and has a
ftopple *p* fitted to its upper mouth,
which has an hole through its middle. The upper veffel C holds juft
half as much as the middle one B;
and the end *t* of the crooked tube,
goes

4

goes no lower than the middle of the
veffel B.

The Procefs.

Fill the middle veffel B with fpring,
or any other clean and wholefome water, and join to it again the upper veffel
C. Pour water into the veffel A (by
the opening *m*, or otherwife) fo as to
cover the rifing part of its bottom.
About three quarters of a pint, or a
little more, will be fufficient. Fill an
ounce phial with oil of vitriol, and add
it to the water, fhaking the veffel fo as
to mix them well together. As heat
is generated, it will be better to add
the oil by a little at a time, otherwife
a hazard is run of breaking the veffel.
Put to this, through a wide glafs, or
paper funnel, about an ounce of powdered raw chalk, or marble*. The
funnel

* White marble being firft granulated, or
pounded like coarfe fand, is much better for the
purpofe

funnel muft be ufed in order to prevent
the powder from touching the infide
of the veffel's mouth ; for if that happen, it will ftick fo ftrongly to the
neck of the veffel B, as not to admit
of their being feparated without breaking. Place immediately the two veffels B and C (faftened to each other)
into the mouth of the veffel A, as in
the figure, and all the fixed air which
is difengaged from the chalk or mar-

purpofe than pounded chalk, becaufe it is harder ;
and therefore the action of the diluted acid upon it
is flower, and lafts a very confiderable time. The
fupply of fixed air from it is therefore much more
regular than with the chalk. In general, it continues to furnifh fixed air more than twenty-four
hours. When no more air is produced, if the water be decanted from the veffel A, and the white
fediment wafhed off, the remaining granulated
marble may be employed again by adding to it frefh
water, and a new quantity of oil of vitriol. A farther produce of fixed air will then be furnifhed,
and this may be repeated until all the marble be
diffolved.

ble

ble by the oil of vitriol, will pafs up
through the valve in S into the veffel
B. When this fixed air comes to the
top of the veffel B, it will diflodge
from thence as much water as is equal
to its bulk; which water will be
forced up through the crooked tube
into the upper veffel C.

Care muft be taken not to fhake
the veffel A when the powdered chalk
is put in ; otherwife a great and fud-
den effervefcence will enfue, which
will perhaps expel part of the contents. In fuch cafe it may be neceffary to open a little the ftopple *m*, in
order to give vent, otherwife the veffel
A may burft. It will be proper alfo
to throw away the contents, and wafh
the veffel ; for the matter will ftick
between the necks of the veffels, and
cement them together. The operation muft then be begun afrefh. But
if the chalk be thrown in without
fhaking

ſhaking the machine, or if marble be.
uſed, the effervefcence will not be
violent. If the chalk be put into the
veffel loofely wrapt up in paper, this
accident will be ftill better guarded
againſt. When the effervefcence goes
on well, the veffel C will foon be filled
with water, and the veffel B half
filled with air ; which will eafily be
known to be the cafe by the air going
up in large bubbles through the
crooked tube *r t.*

When this is obferved, take off the
two veffels B and C together as they
are, and ſhake them ſo that the water
and air within them may be much
agitated. A great part of the fixed
air will be abforbed into the water ;
as will appear by the end of the crooked tube being confiderably under the
furface of the water in the veffel.
The ſhaking them for two or three
minutes will be fufficient for this pur-
poſe.

pofe. Thefe veffels muft not be fhook while joined to the under one A, otherwife too great an effervefcence will be occafioned in the latter; together with the ill confequences abovementioned. After the water and air have been fufficiently agitated, loofen the upper veffel C, fo that the remaining water may fall down into B, and, the unabforbed air pafs out. Put thefe veffels together, and replace them into the mouth of A, in order that B, may be again half filled with fixed air. Shake the veffels B and C, and let out the unabforbed air, as before. By repeating the operation three or four times, the water will be fufficiently impregnated.

Whenever the effervefcence nearly ceafes in the veffel A, it may be renewed by giving it a gentle fhake, fo that the powdered chalk or marble at the bottom may be mixed with the oil

of

of vitriol and water above it; for then a greater quantity of fixed air will be difengaged.

When the effervefcence can be no longer renewed by fhaking the veffel A, either more chalk muft be put in, or more oil of vitriol; or more water, if neither of thefe produce the defired effects.

The ingenious Mr. Magellan has ftill farther improved the contrivance of Dr. Nooth and Mr. Parker. He has two fets of the veffels B and C. While he is fhaking the air and water contained in one of thefe fets, the other may be receiving fixed air from the veffel A. By this means twice the quantity of water may be impregnated in the fame time. He has a wooden ftand K (Fig. 5.) to fix the veffels B C on, when taken off from A, which is very convenient. He has a fmall tin trough for meafuring the quantity

quantity of chalk or marble requifite
for one operation, and a wide glafs
funnel for putting it through into the
veffel A, to prevent its fticking to the
fides, as mentioned before.

He has alfo contrived a ftopple
without an hole to be ufed occafionally
inftead of the perforated one *p*.   It
has a kind of bafon at the top to hold
an additional weight when neceffary.
(See Fig. 6.)   The ftopple muft be
of a conical figure, and very loofe ;
but fo exactly and fmoothly ground as
to be air-tight merely by its preffure,
which may be encreafed by additional
weights put into its bafon.   Its ufe is
tò comprefs the fixed air on the water,
and thereby encreafe the impregnation.   For by keeping the air on the
water in this compreffed ftate, the
latter may be made to fparkle like
Champaign.   And if the veffels be
ftrong,

ftrong, there will be no danger of their burfting in the operation.

If the veffels be fuffered to ftand fix or eight hours, the water will be fufficiently impregnated even without agitation. But by employing the means above defcribed, it may be done in as many minutes.

The water thus impregnated may be drawn out at the opening *k*. But if it be not wanted immediately, it will be better to let it remain in the machine, where it has no communication with the external air. Otherwife the fixed air flies off by degrees, and the water becomes vapid and flat; as alfo happens to other acidulous waters. But it may be kept a long time in bottles well ftopped, efpecially if they be placed with their mouths downwards.

This water is more pleafant to the tafte than the natural Pyrmont or

Seltzer

Seltzer waters ; as, befides their fixed air they contain faline particles of a difagreeable tafte, which are known to contribute little or nothing to their medicinal virtues; and may, in fome cafes, be hurtful. The artificial wa-ter is alfo double the ftrength of the natural; the latter containing fcarce half of the fixed air which can thus be communicated to the former.

N. B. Mr. Blades, of Ludgate-Hill, has ftill further improved this apparatus, by changing the ftopple at *k* for a glafs cock, which is more convenient. He has likewife altered the middle veffel B into a form more advantageous for the impregnation. See Fig. 7. With it are alfo given, a phial for meafuring the vitriolic acid, a tin meafure for the chalk or marble, and a glafs funnel to pafs it through.

A METHOD

A METHOD OF IMITATING THE SULPHUREOUS MINERAL WATERS, BY IMPREGNATING WATER WITH HEPATIC AIR.

We may imitate the *fulphureous* mineral waters, as well as the *acidulous* ones, or thofe impregnated with fixed air. The procefs is fufficiently fimple; and the fame apparatus will ferve for both.

Inftead of limeftone, chalk, or marble, *liver of fulphur* is to be ufed. It may be bought ready prepared of the chymifts or apothecaries; or may eafily be prepared as follows:

Mix together equal parts of brimftone, and of clean pot afhes*, and place them in a crucible, or unglazed difh, over a very gentle fire. Keep them ftirring with a ftick 'till they

* Quick lime may be ufed inftead of pot afhes, taking care to chufe it well burnt.

are

are united together into a blood-red mafs. Put it, while warm, into a bottle, which is to be kept well clofed.

Put a fufficient quantity of this fubftance, with the oil of vitriol and water, into the part A of the apparatus, and proceed as defcribed in the procefs for impregnating water with fixed air; the *hepatic* air will arife; the water in the middle veffel B will be impregnated with it, will fmell ftrongly fulphureous, and refemble the celebrated waters of *Aix la Chapelle,* &c. in the fame manner as thofe impregnated with fixed air refemble thofe of *Pyrmont* and *Seltzer.*

The water thus impregnated may be heated, by putting it into a clofe veffel, placed in one that contains boiling water, and it is then a *warm fulphureous water.*

If it be not ufed immediately, it

E   fhould

fhould be preferved in glafs or ftone bottles, well corked, and cemented and placed with the corks downward in a cellar.

To imitate more exactly the feveral Mineral Waters.

This confifts only in adding to the water to be impregnated, the folid matters which they are found to leave behind on evaporation. For example:

I. PYRMONT WATER.

Add to the water in the middle veffel B, in the proportion of about 30 grains of vitriolated magnefia*, ten grains of common falt, two fcruples of magnefia alba, two fcruples of chalk, and a dram of iron filings, or

---

* Epfom falt, or Sal Catharticus Amarus. In this edition the names of the New London Pharmacopœia are commonly ufed.

iron

iron wire, clean and free from ruft, to one gallon of water, and impregnate the whole with fixed air in the manner defcribed. Let them remain 'till the other ingredients, and as much of the iron as is neceffary, are diffolved, which will be in two or three days.

2. SPA WATER.

Take of natron and magnefia of each a fcruple, of common falt eight grains, water a gallon; impregnate them with fixed air; a few iron filings muft alfo be added.

3. SELTZER WATER.

Take of natron feven fcruples, common falt a dram and half, magnefia one fcruple, water a gallon, and impregnate them with fixed air.

4. SEIDSCUTZ PURGING WATER, (refembling our EPSOM.)

Take of vitriolated magnefia three
E 2 ounces,

ounces, water a gallon, and impregnate them with fixed air.

5. AIX-LA-CHAPELLE WATER.

Take of sea salt two scruples, natron a dram and half, chalk two scruples, water a gallon. Impregnate them with hepatic air, after having first caused them to absorb ninety-six ounce measures of fixed air.

Other waters may in like manner be imitated by adding Epsom salt for purging waters, sea salt for salt waters, &c. And as some waters (as the cold sulphureous ones) contain both *fixed* and *sulphureous* air, a mixture of liver of sulphur and chalk may be put into the vessel A with the oil of vitriol, by which means both these airs will be produced, and the water of course impregnated with them. In making artificial mineral waters, distilled water ought always to be used.

A N

AN

ACCOUNT

OF THE

NATURE, PROPERTIES,

AND

MEDICINAL VIRTUES

OF THE

Principal Mineral Waters

IN

GREAT BRITAIN AND IRELAND;

AND OF THOSE

MOST IN REPUTE IN FOREIGN PARTS.

Digefted into Alphabetical Order.

By JOHN ELLIOT, M. D.

INTRODUCTION.

THE following treatife on mineral waters being intended for the Public in general, the Editor has endeavoured to couch it in fuch terms as that it may be underftood by thofe who are unacquainted with the art of phyfic. Such an account has been judged by many very proper to be fubjoined to the foregoing differtation.

All the mineral waters in *England*, of any note, will be found noticed in this tract: together with their virtues, and the method, and feafon of ufing them, fo far as could be learnt from the authors who have been confulted on the occafion. To thefe are added all the principal mineral waters of *Scotland* and *Ireland*, as well as the moft celebrated ones which the En-

glifh

glifh valetudinarian may have occafion to vifit on the continent.

The greateft part of the books which have hitherto been written on this fubject, abound with experiments tending to fhow the *analyfis* of thofe waters. But this can be of little ufe except to the faculty; and muft be dry, and perfectly uninterefting to common readers. Befides, the neceffity of fuch accounts is fuperceded by fpecifying the ingredients themfelves with which the waters are impregnated, and their virtues as medicines; to fhow which is the fole end of thefe experiments. It would alfo have fwelled the volume to an unwieldy fize. For this laft reafon, as alfo becaufe it was judged wholly unneceffary and fuperfluous, the defcriptions of the places in which the refpective waters are fituated, are likewife omitted.

For

For the convenience of the reader, the waters are arranged in *alphabetical* order, by which means they will the more readily be found. I wonder indeed that this method is not obferved by authors on many other occafions. For though there be a fyftematical arrangement of the things treated of in their books, yet the reader is, after all, obliged to refer to an *index*; which in fact is an alphabetical arrangement of the particulars of the fubject.

The reader will find accounts of a great number of waters which he probably never heard of before. As many of thefe are of fimilar virtues to others which are more famous, the invalid will be inftructed where to find a mineral water proper for his complaint near at hand, when it might not be convenient for him, on account of the diftance, or otherwife,

E 5

to repair to thofe of greater *note,* though perhaps not of fuperior *virtue.*

For this purpofe alfo, as well as for the more readily finding out waters of particular virtues, the waters are alfo claffed or arranged according to their refpective mineral properties; as will prefently be feen.

Water, from the nature of the foil over which it paffes, and other accidents to which it is expofed, is always more or lefs impregnated with foreign particles. According to the nature of thefe particles, the properties of the water are different. Hence we have *hard* water, *foft* water, *falt* water, and the almoft infinite variety of *mineral* waters. The principal of the latter, in this part of the world, will be found noticed in the following tables.

1ft. CHA-

1ſt. CHALYBEATE WATERS.

Hampſtead	Glendy
Carlton	Aberbrothick
Iſlington	Cobham
Leez	Tunbridge
Markſhall	Buxton
Felſtead	Millar's Spa
Wellenbrow	Latham
Ayleſham	Tibſhelf
Malvern	Chippenham
Colurian	Witham
Harrogate	Lancaſter
Road	Whiteacre
Ilmington	Weſt Aſhton
Birmingham	Cawthorp
Cannock	Derby
Moſs Houſe	Weatherſtack
Wigan	Filah
Sene	Dortſhill
Thetford	Stanger
Lincomb	Dunſe
Llandrindod	Caſtle Connel
Peterhead	Tralee

E 6   Granſhaw

Granſhaw	Wexford
Newtown Stewart	Ballyſpellan
Galway	Nezdenice
Coolauran	Kuka
Liſdonvarna	Spa
Ballycaſtle	Zahorovice
Glanmile	Bromley
Kanturk	* Bath
Dunnard	* Matlock.
Maccroomp	

Chalybeate waters are the moſt uſeful and beneficial to health of any of the mineral waters; and are very plentiful in this iſland.

Waters are known to be chalybeate by their ſtriking a reddiſh purple, or black colour with an infuſion of galls; and according to the height of the colour, provided the ſtrength of the infuſion be the ſame, we judge of the ſtrength of the water as a chalybeate.

The iron in thoſe waters is held in ſolution by means of fixed air, as may be judged from what has been already

ſaid

faid on this fubject. As the fixed air
foon flies off on expofing the water,
the iron falls to the bottom in form
of a brownifh yellow powder. Hence
thefe waters ftrike the deepeft black
with galls at the fpring head; and in
time they wholly lofe that property.

They have a brifk acidulous or vinous tafte when frefh, and tinge the
ftools black.

Taken inwardly they ftrengthen
the conftitution in general, increafe
the tone of the fibres, quicken the
circulation, and reftore a proper confiftence to the blood when in a too
thin and watery ftate. And hence
they are found to invigorate the
whole frame. They are good in
difeafes arifing from weaknefs; in
fpafmodic diforders, arifing from too
great irritability and relaxation of the
nervous fyftem; in fluor albus, and
gleets; in female obftructions; in
hyfteric

hyfteric and hypochondriacal diforders; in lofs of appetite and digeftion;
and in a variety of other complaints,
as will be fpecified in treating of the
refpective waters; they differing fomewhat in their virtues.

Previous to a courfe of thefe waters, bleeding, and a cooling purge,
may be neceffary, in cafe of heat and
fever; and coftivenefs fhould alfo be
avoided while drinking them. Where
there is much fever, and alfo in ulcers
of the lungs, and in confirmed obftructions attended with fever, the ufe
of thefe waters is improper.

Patients ought to begin with drinking a fmall quantity of thefe waters
every morning, and gradually to increafe the dofe. A temperate and
moderate diet, and gentle exercife
fhould alfo be obferved while taking
them.

If the water be too cold for the
ftomach,

ftomach, a bottle containing fome of it may be placed in warm water juft before drinking.

Acids, tea, and other things, which decompofe thefe waters, fhould not be taken for fome time before or after drinking them.

Befides iron, thefe waters ufually contain fea falt, natron, a purging falt, or other fubftance, as will be noticed when treating of them.

2d. CHALYBEATE PURGING WA-
TERS.

Knowfley	Thirfk
Burlington	Hartlepool
Aftrope	Thornton
Coventry	Orfton
Bournley	Stenfield
Townley	Kirby
Newham Regis	Tarleton
Binley	Malton
Kingfcliff	Afwarby
	Scarborough

Scarborough	Egra
Cheltenham	Nevil Holt
Bagnigge	Ballycaftle
Stoke	Deddington
Woodham Ferris	Drig-Well
Hanlys	Inglewhite
Athlone	Gainfborough
Mount Pallas	Thorp Arch
Killinfhanvally	Caftlemaign
Cleves	Ballynahinch
Hoff Geifmar	Jeffop
Pyrmont	Driburg.

Thefe chalybeate waters contain a greater proportion of purging falt than of any other folid matter, and therefore when taken in fufficient quantity (feveral pints) they operate by ftool. They have this advantage over other purges, that they do not exhauft the ftrength.

If taken in lefs quantity, as alteratives, they operate chiefly by urine,

and

and then they fall rather under the firſt claſs of theſe waters than the preſent.—*See what was ſaid of chaly-beate waters.*

3d. SULPHUREOUS WATERS.

Sutton Bog	Harrogate
Wigleſworth	Maudſby
Chadlington	Crickleſpaw
Bilton	Broughton
Queen Camel	Shettlewood
Nottington	Reddleſtone
Drumgoon	Durham
Swadlingbar	Wardrow
Derryleſter	Skipton
Liſbeak	Landrindod
Killaſher	Moffat
Mechan	Corſtorphin
Aſhwood	Caſtle Loed
Derryhence	Fairburn
Drumaſnave	Rippon
Anaduff	Groſſenendorf
Aphaloo	* Aix la Chapelle
	* Borſet

* Borſet   * Baden Baden
* Bareges   * Saint Amand.

Waters called *ſulphureous* do not contain an actual ſulphur, but are impregnated with a gas, or ſpirit (the hepatic air already deſcribed) which gives them their ſulphureous ſmell. Beſides this, they uſually contain either natron, ſea ſalt, a purging ſalt, iron, an earth, or other matter, and commonly ſeveral of theſe in different proportions.

Waters of this ſort are diuretic, and ſtrongly diaphoretic, and are therefore good in cutaneous diſeaſes, uſed both internally and externally. They are alſo good in chronic obſtructions; and in diſorders proceeding from acidity, from worms, &c.

They uſually make ſilver appear of a copper colour.

4th. SUL-

4th. SULPHUREOUS PURGING WA-
TERS*.

Aſkeron	Upminſter
Croft	Codſalwood
Cawley	Wirkſworth
Cunley Houſe	Derrindaff
Buglawton	Owen Bruen
Loanſbury	Pettigoe
Normanby	Enghien
Shapmoor	

Theſe waters differ from thoſe in the preceding claſs in containing a purging ſalt as the principal ſolid ingredient, and therefore operating by ſtool. They are good in the ſame diſorders as the alterative ſulphureous waters, as alſo for foulneſſes of the bowels, &c.

* Some of the chálybeate purging waters are alſo ſulphureous.

5th. ACI-

5th. ACIDULOUS, OR SALINE WA-
TERS.

Seltzer	Cape Clare
Tilbury	Buch
Clifton	Tonftein
Glaftonbury	* Mount d'Or
Toberbony	* Chaude Fontaine
Carrickmore	* Pifa.
St. Bartholomew	

The waters of this clafs contain
natron. This falt, as the waters are
taken up from the fountain, is fatu-
rated, or rather fuperfaturated, with
fixed air; hence the waters do not
then manifeft any alkaline quality; on
the contrary, they curdle with foap,
and are termed *acidulæ*. This *fixed
air*, or *aërial acid*, however, being
very volatile, foon exhales when the
water is heated, or ftands awhile expofed, and then the alkali manifefts
itfelf.

The

The general virtues of thefe waters may be known from what is faid in the alphabet, under the article SELT-ZER WATER.

6. SALINE PURGING WATERS.

Barrowdale	Acton
Leamington	Epfom
New Cartmal, or	Alkerton
Rougham	Ball, or Bandwell
St. Erafmus	Llandrindod
Cargyrle	Kenfington
Dortfhill	Richmond
Alford	Upminfter
Dulwich	Seidlitz
Holt	* Balaruc
Stretham	Sea Water
Kilburn	Dog and Duck
Moreton-fee	Kinalton
Hanlys	Brentwood
Conmer	Colchefter
Bagnigge	Sydenham
Barnet	Carrickfergus
North-hall	* Bagniers.

Thefe

Thefe waters are impregnated with fea falt, and alfo with a purging falt. This, which has formerly received various names from different authors, is now generally fuppofed to be *vitriolated magnefia:* though, from difference of figure and folubility, many incline to think, that there may be different purging falts in different, or even in the fame waters. They who hold the former opinion, attribute this diverfity of appearance to a combination with different ingredients.

They differ in ftrength; fome of them purge fufficiently in the quantity of a pint; while two, three, four, five, or fix pints of others are neceffary to produce that effect. Some again are fo weak as to require the addition of fome other purgative falt.

Given in fmall quantities they act as diuretics and alteratives.

They

They are good in fcrophulous and fcorbutic complaints, ulcers, and other difeafes which make their appearance on the fkin, and are likewife ufed as baths, and fomentations in thefe and other diforders.

The virtues of the preceding clafs of waters depend in a great meafure on the prefence of their *fixed air*. The waters of the prefent clafs feem to derive their virtues principally from the faline matters which they contain.

7. VITRIOLIC WATERS.

Shadwell	Hartfel
Weftwood	Crofs-town
Swanzy	Nobber
Haigh	Cafhmore
Vahls	Kilbrew.

Thefe waters are impregnated with green vitriol or copperas, and ftrike a black colour with galls.

They are chiefly ufed outwardly
for

for wafhing old fores and the like,
and frequently with good effect. In
fome cafes, however, they are taken
inwardly in fmall dofes, and then they
prove emetic and purgative.

8. WATERS WHICH CONTAIN AN EARTH.

Newton-dale	* Briftol
Bale	* Buxton
Knarefborough	* Mallow.
Glavely	

The cold waters of this clafs have
a petrifying quality. The virtues of
the waters of this clafs being different,
the reader is referred to the refpective
articles in the alphabet for an account
of them.

The above arrangement of mineral
waters is intended more for the convenience of the reader not verfed in
phyfic, than as a *fyftematical* one.

Had the latter idea been adopted, it
would

would have been neceffary perhaps to have made a divifion of the waters into *hot* and *cold*, in imitation of the learned Dr. Donald Monro; from whofe ingenious work, together with thofe of Dr. Short, Dr. Rutty, and a few others, the following treatife has been chiefly compiled*.

There are a great number of *cold* mineral waters in England; but the number of the *hot* ones is very fmall. In the above catalogue, the *latter* are diftinguifhed from the *former* by having an ASTERISK placed before them. Thofe of greateft note on the continent, however, are alfo noticed; in many parts of which they abound.

The caufe of the heat of thofe waters is, in fome inftances, fubterraneous fire; as is the cafe with fome

---

* The quantity of waters to be drank, and fome other particulars, are not always mentioned by authors, but they may eafily be learnt on the fpot.

F　　　　which

which are fituated near volcanos. In other cafes the heat arifes from the mineral ingredients with which they are impregnated in their paffage. And the fame may be faid of thofe waters which are *cooler* than the common temperature of the atmofphere. Thus it is known, that quick-lime, the pyrites ftone, and other fubftances, thrown into water will-make it *warm.* On the contrary, falts of various kinds make it *colder* than before.

The *warm* waters poffefs many of the virtues and properties of *cold* waters of the fame clafs, and which are impregnated in the fame manner; but they are preferable in many cafes, as from their warmth they are more kindly and agreeable to the ftomachs of weak people, and promote perfpiration.

The warm waters are alfo ufed as

warm

warm baths, and may in general be confidered as warm medicated baths; and thefe by relaxing the fibres, are of ufe in a variety of diforders which take their rife from rigidity, and from fpafm, as alfo from other caufes. Hence their great ufe in rheumatifms, inflammations, coftivenefs, &c. The cure is ufually affifted by the internal ufe of thofe waters at the time.

For complaints of a particular part of the body, either the part is foment-ed with the warm water, or the water is raifed to an height by pumps, or otherwife, and then let fall with force on the difeafed part; this is called *pumping* by the Englifh; the French term it the *Douche*.

Contrivances are alfo ufed for raifing thefe waters into *vapour* or *fleam*, and confining it fo that it may be applied to the whole body, or to particular parts. Thefe contrivances are called *vapour baths*.

Baths are likewife made of the mud found at the bottom of thefe waters; and they have been found ferviceable in removing pains, and achs; and paralytic, and other complaints. The mud is either rubbed on the part, or the part is immerfed in it, as may be judged convenient or proper; when it is collected in quantity in a refervoir for thefe-purpofes, it is called the *mud bath*.

The cold waters are alfo, in fome cafes, ufed externally.

I fhall conclude this introduction by mentioning fome of the moft obvious methods of analyzing, or difcovering the nature of mineral waters.

The various fubftances occafionally found united with water, and with each other by diffufion, or by chemical

cal folution, may be comprifed chiefly, as Dr. Fothergill obferves, under four claffes.

1. AERIAL. Atmofpheric, vital, fixed, inflammable, hepatic, and phlogifticated airs.

2. SALINE. Vitriolic, nitrous, and marine acids; natron, kali, ammonia, and fulphurated kali.

3. METALLIC. Iron, copper, zinc, manganefe, arfenic.

4. EARTHY. Magnefia, lime, clay, barytes, filiceous earth.

Of neutral falts we find the vitriolic acid united with natron, kali, lime, magnefia, clay, iron, copper, and zinc. The nitrous acid with the four former of thefe. The marine acid with the fame; and fometimes with barytes, manganefe, and clay. And the aerial acid with thefe, and

alfo

alfo with iron, zinc, and manganefe.

Sulphur, foffil oil, and extracts from vegetable and animal fubftances, are alfo found fometimes in mineral waters.

From thefe all the virtues of mineral waters are derived, if we except what they obtain from their temperature. To inveftigate them by an accurate analyfis, fome care and attention are neceffary. The following methods are collected from the beft writers on that fubject.

Previous to the chemical examination the fenfible qualities of the water, as tafte, fmell, colour, and degree of tranfparency, fhould be obferved. Thefe, with the fpecific gravity, temperature, and furrounding foil, will afford confiderable information, and point out the readieft methods of analyzing it.

To

To the *tafte* the aerial acid gives a gentle fmartnefs or poignancy : vitriolic or nitrous falts, a bitternefs : lime or felenite, a flight aufterity : alum, a fweetifh aftringency : natron, and marine falt, a naufeous brackifh-nefs : copper, a flight tafte of brafs : iron, an inky tafte.

To the *fmell* aerial acid exhibits an agreeable penetrating odour like that of fermenting liquors : hepatic air *, an odour like that of a foul gun, or ignited gunpowder.

A brown, reddifh, or yellow *colour*, betrays various impurities : a whitifh indicates clay : a blue, vitriol of copper : a green or variegated film, vitriol of iron ; and this laft is confirmed if there be a yellow ochry fediment.

The examination ought to be made

* A bituminous or afphaltic air gives a fmell fomewhat fimilar to this.

in

in the different feafons, at different times of the day, and particularly in different ftates of the atmofphere, as thefe have confiderable influence on waters.

There are three modes of analyzing mineral waters : by REAGENTS; by EVAPORATION; by DISTILLATION. All thefe have their ufes.

A great number of different re-agents have been employed, of which the following are the principal, and perhaps all that deferve to be noticed.

SYRUP OF VIOLETS. All vegetable blues turn red with acids; green, with alkalis. This has been moft commonly ufed, but many are now difpofed to rejeft it in favour of others. It will fometimes change green with iron ; which, if it were trufted to alone, might lead to miftakes.

TINC-

Tincture of turnsole, or a blue tincture prepared from lacmofs, appears to be a more fenfible teft; and

The juice of red cabbage, recommended by Mr. Watt, may be in fome cafes preferable to either.

Infusion of Brazil wood, which is red, with alkalis becomes blue. Acids change it yellow, and reftore the red deftroyed by an alkali. Paper ftained with the infufion, a little ftarch being previoufly boiled in it, is a more fenfible teft than the infufion itfelf.

Infusion of turmeric is made brown by alkalis.

Tincture of galls in fpirit of wine. This fhould be made as ftrong as poffible. It readily difcovers iron, in proportion to the quantity of which it will vary in colour through different gradations of purple, and if the quan-

F 5   tity

tity be large it will appear quite black.

PHLOGISTICATED, or as it is now more generally called, PRUSSIAN ALKALI, is alſo uſed as a teſt of iron, with which it exhibits Pruſſian blue. It precipitates copper of a reddiſh brown colour; zinc and manganeſe, white; but theſe two precipitates may be diſtinguiſhed from each other by the latter becoming black by calcination, which effects no change in the former : it likewiſe precipitates other metals. An improved method of preparing this alkali may be found in the firſt volume of the Analytical Review.

CONCENTRATED VITRIOLIC ACID. It diſcovers barytes.

FUMING NITROUS ACID is recommended by Bergman to precipitate ſulphur, when the water contains it in the form of hepar.

ACID CF SUGAR is a very fenſible teſt

teſt of lime, but does not always detect it, being incapable of difengaging
it when held in folution by a confiderable excefs of any acid, the fparry
and acetous excepted. This is a curious fact not generally known.

FIXED VEGETABLE ALKALI precipitates all earths, except barytes and
metals. M. de Fourcroy recommends
it to be perfectly pure, or cauftic; but
obferves, that it will in that ftate precipitate any lefs foluble neutral falt
with an alkaline bafe.

VOLATILE ALKALI. This, if
perfectly pure, decompofes only earthy
falts with bafes of clay or magnefia;
but if aerated, will alfo decompofe calcareous falts by double affinity. It
changes water containing copper
blue.

LIME WATER detects the prefence
of aerial acid, with which it forms a
precipitate. As thirty-two parts of
chalk

chalk contain thirteen of the aerial acid, the quantity of the latter, in a mineral water, may be afcertained by the weight of the chalk depofited. It alfo decompofes metallic falts, and clay or magnefia when united with the marine or vitriolic acids.

SALITED BARYTES is a moft fenfible teft of vitriolic acid, taking it from every other bafe, and forming with it an infoluble compound.

NITRATED SILVER, when diffolved in diftilled water, will detect the fmalleft veftige of a marine acid : but it is by no means an accurate teft, as vitriolic acid, if in confiderable quantity, occafions alfo a precipitate with it ; and the fame effect is ftill more evidently produced by fixed alkali, chalk, or magnefia, unlefs nitrous acid fufficient to faturate them be previoufly added.

NITRATED MERCURY. Of this there

there are two kinds, one made with heat, the other without. Many circumftances combine to render this an extremely fallacious teft.

A SOLUTION OF ARSENIC in the marine acid will precipitate fulphur from water in which it is held diffolved by means of fixed air.

We may add, that WHITE ARSE-NIC becomes yellow if immerfed in water containing hepatic gas : and a piece of polifhed iron will receive a copper-colour from water in which copper is diffolved. By the latter method copper has been detected in pine-apple rum, in which the aqua ammoniæ produced no change.

The examination of mineral waters has generally been made with too fmall quantities. The beft method is to mix feveral pounds with each reagent, till the latter ceafes to pro-

duce

duce any precipitate. It fhould then be fuffered to fubfide for twenty-four hours in a well-covered veffel, and, after being filtered, the precipitate may be weighed and examined.

Evaporation is the fecond means employed for obtaining the fixed principles of a mineral water. For this purpofe a large quantity fhould be employed; fometimes even feveral hundred pounds. Veffels of metal fhould by no means be ufed. The beft methods are, evaporating to drynefs in open glafs veffels in the waterbath, or, which is preferable, in glafs retorts in a fand-bath.

The refiduum thus obtained is to be weighed, and put into a phial with three or four times its weight of fpirit of wine. The phial being well fhaken, it fhould be fet by for fome hours to fubfide. What the fpirit will.

will not diffolve, being dried, fhould
be mixed with eight times its weight
of cold diftilled water, weighing it
again previoufly to afcertain the quantity taken up by the fpirit. What is
not foluble in this proportion of cold
water, fhould be boiled in four or five
hundred times its weight of the fame
fluid. All thefe products, with the
refiduum of the latter, are to be examined feparately.

The fpirituous folution will contain calcareous and magnefian muriate. After evaporating to drynefs,
the refiduum is to be diffolved in water. Add to this vitriolic acid: the
calcareous earth will precipitate in
the form of felenite, and the magnefian may be obtained in that of Epfom
falt, from which kali will precipitate
the magnefia.

The cold water will have diffolved
the neutral falts with alkaline or earthy
bafes,

bafes, and fometimes a fmall quantity of martial vitriol. As a greater or lefs number of thefe are almoft always mixed, and in various proportions, fome care is neceffary to afcertain them. They fhould be feparated, if practicable, by a flow evaporation. In this way they make their appearance according to their promptitude to cryftallize. But as this method does not always fucceed perfectly, however careful we may be in conducting the evaporation, it will be neceffary to re-examine the falts obtained at the different periods of the procefs. Alkaline falt is known by its lixivious tafte and effervefcence with acids. Diftilled vinegar will determine whether this be vegetable or mineral, as with the former it yields a deliquefcent falt; with the latter, foliated cryftals. Neutral falts compofed of vitriolic acid may be decompofed by

the

the falited barytes. The vitriolic acid
will decompofe thofe into which the
nitrous or marine acid enters : if it be
the former, red fumes will arife ; if
the latter, grey. The bafes of falts
compounded of the vitriolic acid may
be diftinguifhed by the figure of the
cryftals, except natron and magnefia;
but the latter renders lime-water turbid, the former does not. If the acid
be the marine, acid of tartar will take
from it kali, and a true tartar will
be precipitated : if it be united with
natron, no decompofition will enfue.
The vitriolic acid will take from it
calcareous earth, and form felenite ;
or magnefia, and form Epfom falt ;
or clay, and form alum. If copper be
the bafis, aqua ammoniæ will render
the folution blue ; if iron, tincture of
galls will turn it purple or black.
Cretaceous foda, if there be any, is
ufually depofited with the muriatic
falts :

falts : they may be feparated, however, by the following procefs of
M. Gioanetti.   Wafh the mixed falt
with diftilled vinegar :   dry it and
pour on fpirit of wine :   this will diffolve the acetous foda, without act-
ing on the marine falt.   By evaporation and calcination the foda will be
left pure, and thus its quantity accu-
rately determined.

If the water took up any thing during the boiling, in the third procefs,
it muft be felenite.   This the pure
kali will precipitate.

The refiduum, on which neither
the fpirit of wine nor the water could
act, may confift of calcareous earth,
aerated magnefia or iron, clay and
quartz.   The two laft are rare.   A
brown or yellow colour indicates
iron ;   a white grey, the abfence of it.
If it contain iron, it fhould be moif-
tened and expofed to the rays of the

§   fun,

fun, and, when the iron is perfectly
rufted, digefted in diftilled vinegar.
This will diffolve the lime and magnefia, which may be feparated by the
vitriolic acid, as we have pointed out
above. The iron and clay are foluble in pure marine acid, from which
the former may be precipitated by the
Pruffian alkali; the latter, by the
mild vegetable alkali. The matter
which remains is ufually quartzofe:
this the blowpipe will afcertain.

DISTILLATION is employed to
procure the aeriform fluids contained
in water. For this purpofe fome
pounds muft be put into a retort, of
which they fhould not fill more than
half or two thirds: to the retort a
recurved tube is to be adapted, paff-
ing underneath an inverted veffel
filled with mercury. The retort is
then to be heated till the water boils,

or

or till no more elaſtic fluid paſſes over.
Hepatic air, and fixed air, are thoſe
moſt commonly met with in waters.
The former is eaſily diſtinguiſhable
by its peculiar ſmell; the latter by
being abſorbed by lime-water, from
which it precipitates the calcareous
earth.

AN

ACCOUNT

OF THE

MEDICINAL VIRTUES, *&c.*

OF

MINERAL WATERS.

ABCOURT, *near St. Germains, four leagues from Paris.*

IT is a brisk chalybeate water, impregnated with fixed air, and natron; and resembles the waters of *Spa* and *Ilmington*.

ABERBROTHOCK, *in Scotland.*

It is a chalybeate water, similar to those of *Peterhead* and *Glendy*.

ACTON,

A C T O N, *near London, in the county of Middlefex.*

The wells are much frequented in May, June, and July.

The water is clear, and without fmell, but its tafte is fomewhat bitterifh.

It contains upwards of five drams of vitriolated magnefia in the gallon.

It is one of the ftrongeft purging waters about London; and is noted for caufing a great forenefs in the fundament.

A G H A L O O, or A P H A L O O, *in the county of Tyrone, Ireland.*

It is a fulphureous water of the fame kind with that of *Swadlingbar,* but ftronger. Like that, it is alfo impregnated with natron, and a fmall quantity of purging falt.

AIX-

Aix-la-Chapelle*, *in the* duchy *of* Juliers, *Germany.*

This place has long been famous for its hot fulphureous waters and

* My friend, the ingenious Dr. Simmons, F. R. S. who made many experiments on the waters during his refidence at this place, has favoured me with an account of their feveral temperatures, as repeatedly obferved by himfelf, with a thermometer conftructed by Nairne.

The fpring which fupplies the Emperor's bath
  (Bain de l'Empereur), the New Bath *(Bain Neuf)*, and the Queen of Hungary's bath
  (Bain de la Reine de Hongrie) — 127°
St. Quirin's bath *(Bain de St. Quirin)* 112°
The Rofe bath *(Bain de la Rofe)*, and the
  Poor's bath *(Bain des Pauvres)*, both which
  are fupplied by the fame fpring — 112°
Charles's bath *(Bain de Charles)*, and St.
  Corneille's bath *(Bain de St. Corneille)* 112°
The fpring ufed for drinking is in the High
  Street, oppofite to Charles's bath; the heat
  of it at the pump is —— —— 106°

Dr. Afh makes the greateft heat 136° of Fahrenheit, placing the temperatures of the different baths from 3° to 9° higher than in the above account.

baths.

baths. They arife from feveral fources,
which fupply eight baths conftructed
in different parts of the town.

Thefe waters near the fources are
clear and pellucid, and have a ftrong
fulphureous fmell refembling the
wafhings of a foul gun; but they
lofe this fmell by expofure to air.
Their tafte is faline, bitter, and urinous. They do not contain iron.
They are alfo neutral near the fountain, but afterwards are manifeftly,
and pretty ftrongly alkaline, infomuch
that cloaths are wafhed with them
without foap.

The gallon contains about two
fcruples of fea falt, the fame quantity of
chalk, and a dram and half of natron.

They are at firft naufeous and harfh,
but by habit become familiar and
agreeable. At firft drinking alfo they
generally affect the head.

Their general operation is by ftool
and

and urine, without griping or diminution of ſtrength ; and they alſo promote perſpiration.

The quantity to be drunk as an alterative, is to be varied according to the conſtitution, and other circumſtances of the patient. In general, it is beſt to begin with a quarter, or half a pint in the morning, and increaſe the doſe afterwards to pints, as may be found convenient. The water is beſt drunk at the fountain. When it is required to purge, it ſhould be drunk in large and often repeated draughts.

In regard to bathing, this alſo muſt be determined by the age, ſex, ſtrength, &c. of the patient, and by the ſeaſon. The degree of heat of the bath ſhould likewiſe be conſidered. The tepid ones are in general the beſt, though there are ſome caſes in which the hotter ones are moſt pro-

G   per.

per.   But even in thefe it is beft to
begin with the temperate baths, and
increafe the heat gradually.

Thefe waters are efficacious in difeafes proceeding from indigeftion, and
from foulnefs of the ftomach and
bowels. In rheumatifms; in the
fcurvy, fcrophula, and difeafes of
the fkin ; in hyfteric, and hypochondriacal diforders ; in nervous complaints and melancholy ; in the ftone
and gravel ; in paralytic complaints ;
in thofe evils which follow an inju-
dicious ufe of mercury, and in many
other cafes.

They ought not however to be given in hectic cafes where there is
heat and fever, in putrid diforders,
or where the blood is diffolved, or the
conftitution much broken down.

ALFORD,

ALFORD, or AWFORD, *in Somer-*
fetfhire, about 24 *miles fouthward*
of Bath.

This falt fpring was difcovered in
1670, from the pigeons which flew
thither in great numbers to drink the
water : thofe birds being known to be
fond of falt.

It contains a purging falt, together
with a portion of fea falt.

It is ftrongly purgative.

It is recommended as cooling,
cleanfing, and attenuating. As a
good remedy in the fcurvy, jaundice,
and other glandular obftruftions. It
alfo promotes urine and fweat, and
therefore is good in gravelly and other
diforders of the kidnies and bladder;
and in complaints arifing from ob-
ftrufted perfpiration.

ALKERTON, *in Gloucefterfhire, near the city of Gloucefter.*

It is a purging water, of the nature of thofe of *Dulwich* and *Epfom.*

ANADUFF, *in the county of Leitrim, Ireland.*

It is a fulphureous water, of the fame kind with thofe of *Killafher* and *Drumafnave,* but weaker.

ANTONIAN.

See *Tonftein.*

ASHWOOD, *in the county of Fermanagh, Ireland.*

It is a fulphureous water; and contains natron, with a fmall quantity of purging falt.

In its virtues it refembles the waters of *Drumgoon* and *Swadlingbar.*

ASKERON,

ASKERON, *five miles from Don-caster, in Yorkshire.*

It is a ftrong fulphureous water, and is flightly impregnated with a purging falt.

A gallon contains forty-eight grains of vitriolated magnefia, with a little fea falt, and a dram and half of earth.

It is recommended internally and externally in ftrumous and other ul-cers, fcabies, leprofy, and fimilar com-plaints.

It is good in chronic obftruétions, and in cafes of worms and foulnefs of the bowels.

It operates by ftool and urine.

ASTROPE, *near Banbury, in Ox-fordfhire.*

It is a brifk, fpirituous, pleafant-tafted chalybeate water, and is alfo gently purgative.

It

It fhould be drunk from three to five quarts in the forenoon.

It is recommended as excellent in female obftructions, the gravel, hypochondria, and fimilar diforders.

A s w a r b y, *feven miles from Grantham, in Lincolnfhire.*

It is a fine blueifh chalybeate water, and is gently laxative without occafioning griping or faintnefs, or a pain in the fundament; which is a common effect of waters impregnated with fea falt. In its virtues it refembles the *Cheltenham* water.

A t h l o n e, *in the county of Rofcommon, Ireland.*

It is a chalybeate water, without colour or fmell, but it will not keep.

It operates by urine, and is gently laxative. It feems to refemble the *Hartlepool* water.

A y l e-

A Y L E S H A M, *in Norfolk.*

It is a flight chalybeate water, fimilar to that of *Iflington.*

B A D E N, *in Auftria, Germany.*

The waters are warm and fulphureous, and have been recommended in thofe diforders in which the *Bareges* and *Aix-la-Chapelle* waters have been found ferviceable. They are particularly fpoken of for the cure of gun-fhot wounds, and the complaints which remain after them.

B A D E N   B A D E N, *in Swabia, Germany.*

There are a number of hot fulphureous fprings and baths in and near this place, which have the fame general virtues as thofe of *Aix-la-Chapelle* and *Bareges.* Taken inwardly they are alfo gently laxative.

B A G-

BAGNERES, *in the Bigorre, France.*

At this place are a variety of warm baths, which are ufed in the fame diforders as thofe of *Aix-la-Chapelle.*

The waters of fome fprings taken internally are diuretic, and others purgative.

BAGNIGGE WELLS PURGING WATER.

It is fituated on the north-eaft fide of London, near Iflington, and is much frequented in the fpring.

It is a falt purging water, containing in the gallon 257 grains of fea falt and vitriolated magnefia mixed.

Its virtues are fimilar to thofe of Pancras and Acton.

The dofe is from a pint to a quart. But it is ufually quickened with Glauber's, or other falts.

The

The CHALYBEATE WATER.

It is clear when it comes from the pump, and has a flight irony tafte.

When firft taken to the quantity of three or four glaffes, it is ufually purgative. But this effect does not continue after the inteftines are cleared of their vitiated contents.

In its virtues it refembles the *Orfton* and other fimilar chalybeates.

BALARUC, *in Languedoc, France.*

The waters of this place are hot, and gently purgative. They have been ufed in many diforders for which falt purging waters are prefcribed.

They contain calcareous and magnefian muriate, fea falt, and chalk.

As they are hot, they have alfo been found particularly ufeful in cafes where warm baths are proper, to affift the operation of fuch waters.

Hence

Hence they have been found particularly ufeful in palfies and rheumatifms, in fcrophula, and many other
diforders.

B A L E M O R E.

See *Ilmington.*

B A L L, or B A N D-W E L L, *in Lin-colnfhire.*

It refembles the *Dropping-Well* water. Four or five half pints are reckoned a fufficient dofe.

BALLYCASTLE, *in Antrim, Ireland.*

It is a chalybeate water, fomewhat
of the nature of thofe of *Iflington* and
Hampftead; only it is flightly fulphureous.

BALLYNAHINCH, *in Down, Ireland.*

It is a very clear, cold, chalybeate
and

and fulphureous water, and is good in fcorbutic and cutaneous difeafes, in lofs of appetite, &c.

BALLYSPELLAN, *near Kilkenny, in Ireland.*

It is a flight chalybeate water, fimilar to thofe of *Iflington* and *Hampftead.*

BAREGES, *in the Bigorre, France.*

There are feveral fprings of hot fulphureous water at this place, which form four baths *.

The water is at firft clear; but by ftanding throws up a thin pellicle, refembling a fine light oil. It has a flight fulphureous fmell, like that of eggs boiled hard. It has a foft and

* Dr. Simmons informs me, that on plunging his thermometer into the hotteft fpring the mercury rofe to 112°.

Dr. Afh placed the hotteft at 122°, the leaft hot at 97°.

fome-

fomewhat naufeous tafte, and feels foft, like foap-water, or oil. Its volatile parts fly off on expofure to the air; and it is beft drunk at the fountain head.

It contains fulphurated kali, with a very fmall portion of fea falt, natron, calcareous earth, and felenite.

This water operates by perfpiration, and by urine; but feldom by ftool. The dofe is ufually a quart, or three pints.

It is alfo ufed as a bath; as a fomentation; and as a douche.

The Barèges waters have been recommended in a variety of diforders; in rheumatifms, palfies, convulfions, cutaneous eruptions, the gout, fcurvy, &c. Alfo in wounds, ulcers, hard tumours; and they are faid to have been efficacious in old gun-fhot wounds, and in hard knots in the urethra after venereal complaints.

B A R-

BARNET and NORTH-HALL.

The *former* fpring is fituated at Eaft Barnet in Hertfordfhire.

The *latter* lies about three miles north of High Barnet.

They are both purging waters, fomewhat of the nature of *Epfom* water, but much weaker. That of *Barnet* is the ftrongeft of the two, containing five drams of vitriolated magnefia, with a little fea falt, in the gallon.

BARROWDALE. *The fpring is about three miles from Kefwick in Cumberland.*

It is a falt water, and much of the nature of that of the fea.

A gallon affords feven ounces and two drams of fea falt mixed with a little vitriolated magnefia.

It is a brifk and rough purge even
to

to ſtrong conſtitutions, occaſioning
great thirſt, and heating the body. A
pint is uſually ſufficient for a doſe.

Taken in leſs quantity (half, or a
quarter of a pint) it operates by urine.

It is of excellent uſe in ſcorbutic
complaints, in the King's evil, and
the leproſy. It is alſo powerful in
removing chronic obſtructions ; in
clearing the blood of acrimonious humours ; in diſeaſes of the ſkin ; and
in all thoſe complaints in which ſea
water is ſerviceable. Like that alſo
it may be uſed externally by way of
fomentation or bath. See *Sea Water*.

BATH, *in Somerſetſhire.*

This place has long been famous
for its warm chalybeate waters. There
are ſeveral ſprings, but their waters
are all of the ſame nature. There
are ſix baths ; but the principal are
the

the *King*'s bath, the *Queen*'s bath, and the *Crofs* bath. The others are only appendages to thefe. The two former raife the thermometer to 116°, the latter to 112°.

The water when viewed in the baths has a greenifh, or fea colour: but in a vial it appears quite tranf-parent and colourlefs, and it fparkles in the glafs.

It has a very flight faline, bitterifh, and chalybeate tafte, which is not dif-agreeable, and fometimes fomewhat of a fulphureous fmell; but this lat-ter is not ufually perceivable, except when the baths are filling.

The gallon of Bath water contains twenty-three grains of chalk, the fame quantity of muriate of magnefia, thirty-eight of fea falt, and 8.1 of aerated iron.

As it rifes from the pump, it con-tains fixed air, or other volatile acid,

in

in a fufficient quantity to curdle milk and diffolve iron.

The Bath water operates powerfully by urine, and promotes perfpiration. If drank quickly, in large draughts, it fometimes purges; but if taken flowly and in fmall quantity, it rather has the contrary effect. An heavinefs of the head, and inclination to fleep, are often felt on firft drinking it.

This water when taken inwardly gives a brifk ftimulus to the nerves and fibres, and feems to give new life and vigour to the whole frame. It alfo powerfully corrects putrefcent acrimony. Hence when taken into the ftomach it is faid to dilute and blunt whatever putrefcent humours it meets with; while its brifk, volatile, chalybeate principles ftimulate and increafe the tone of the ftomach and bowels, and brace up their fibres and nerves.

nerves. Entering the circulation,
they pervade the minuteſt veſſels; dilute, blunt, and correct thoſe fluids
in the blood which are too putreſcent;
increaſe the action of the whole vaſ-
cular ſyſtem to promote the circulation through the ſmalleſt veſſels, to
break down groſs humours, to remove obſtructions, and to promote
ſecretions of the ſkin and kidnies,
for carrying off thoſe fluids that are
unfit to circulate longer in the general
maſs. And hence it is that they have
been found ſo ſerviceable in ſuch a
variety of diſorders. In female complaints, for example; ſuch as obſtructions of the menſes; barrenneſs
proceeding from obſtruction and relaxation of the womb; the fluor albus, &c. In hyſteric and hypochondriacal diſorders; in complaints of
the ſtomach and bowels proceeding
from weakneſs and laxity, or from
putreſ-

putrefcent humours. In pains of the ftomach, attended with bad digeftion, and in many cholicky and other diforders of the ftomach and bowels. In diforders of the head and nerves; fuch as palfies, epilepfies, convulfions, &c. In difeafes of the fkin; the fea fcurvy; leprofy. In obftructions of the liver, fpleen, and other bowels; in gouty and rheumatic complaints; in the ftone and gravel; and in many other difeafes.

Thefe waters being of an heating nature, it is ufual, previous to a courfe of them, to cool the body by gentle purges, by a low diet, and, if found neceffary, by bleeding.

They may be drunk from half a pint, to two, three, or four pints in a day, according to circumftances. The beft method is to take one, two, three, or four half glaffes at proper intervals in the morning; a glafs or two an hour before

before dinner; and as much about the fame time before fupper. The patient in the mean time fhould live upon a light diet, eafy of digeftion; ufe proper exercife; go early to bed; and rife betimes in the morning.

In fome cafes, however, thefe waters are hurtful. In hectic fevers, for example; in fuppurations of the lungs; in fits of the gout; and in the rheumatifm if inflammatory; and indeed in all cafes of inflammation; as alfo where the action of the fibres is already too ftrong, the animal heat too great, and the blood thick and fizy.

The quantity of the waters drank in a day fhould be gradually encreafed to as much as the patient can bear; and after continuing that quantity a fufficient time, it fhould be as regularly diminifhed. The courfe may
be

be continued for a month or fix weeks.

The ufual feafon for the Bath waters is in April, May, and June; and in Auguft, September, and October.

Thefe waters are alfo ufed externally in a variety of diforders, and with good effect, either by bathing or pumping, as occafion may require; efpecially if ufed inwardly at the fame time. Forefts of crutches left there, are an ample teftimony of the efficacy of bathing in paralytic cafes. By foftening and relaxing the parts, and at the fame time giving a gentle ftimulus, they are alfo of fervice in removing many inveterate gouty and rheumatic complaints. In difeafes of the limbs, &c. arifing from obftructions; in fprained, relaxed, and ftiff joints; in fcorbutic and cutaneous difeafes, old fores and ulcers, and in many other cafes; and when the

com-

complaint is local, pumping is generally preferred to bathing.

It is a certain effect of thefe and
other baths, to throw out a rednefs
and kind of eruption on the fkin, efpecially in thofe who are fcorbutic,
&c. But this effect difappears by
their continued ufe, and the diforders
themfelves are at length cured.

The mud and fcum of thefe waters
have alfo been applied with good effect by way of poultice in hard fwellings, in weak joints, in contractions
of the limbs, in fcald heads, running
ulcers, &c. and herbs are fometimes
boiled with them in the Bath water
to a proper confiftence, for thefe and
the like purpofes.

B I L T O N, *near Knarefborough, York
fhire.*

The water has a ftrong fulphureous
fmell,

fmell, and taftes fomewhat faltifh. It
is colder than common water.

It contains natron, with a little
fea falt.

It acts as a gentle purge; and is
fomewhat fimilar in virtue to the *Sutton Bog* water.

BINLEY, *near Coventry, Warwickfhire.*

It is a chalybeate water, and alfo
purgative and diuretic.   It refembles
the *Scarborough* water, but is lefs purgative.

BIRMINGHAM, *in Warwickfhire.*

Near this place is a brifk chalybeate water, which feems to refemble
that of *Hampftead* in *Middlefex.*

BORDS-

BORDSCHEIT, or BORSET*, *about a mile and half from Aix-la-Cha-pelle, Germany.*

The waters are warm, and of the nature of thofe of Aix-la-Chapelle, being, however, fomewhat more pur-gative; but they are only ufed as baths, for the difeafes in which the waters laft mentioned are recommended, and alfo in dropfical and oedematous cafes.

BRABACH, *in the diftrict of Men-gerfkirchen, in the county of Naf-fau, Germany.*

It is a brifk fpirity chalybeate wa-ter, which may be preferved long in

* The waters at this place, which is only about a mile from Aix-la-Chapelle, are diftinguifhed into the upper and lower fprings. The former, which contain no hepatic air, were found by Dr. Simmons to raife the thermometer to 158°; the latter, all of which are fulphureous, to 127° only. All the baths are fupplied by the firft.

§   well-

well-ftopt bottles, though it foon
fpoils in the open air. It has a fomewhat falt, fulphureous, and aftringent
tafte, and contains natron.

It refembles the German *Spa Water*
in its general virtues.

B R A N D O L-A, *in Italy.*

It is a flight chalybeate water, extremely limpid and cryftalline, impregnated with an alkaline falt, and
abounding in fixed air. It fmells
fomewhat fulphureous, and has an
acidulous tafte.

It is commonly drunk from two
pints to a gallon or more in a day. It
promotes urine and perfpiration, and
is gently laxative.

Its virtues feem to refemble thofe
of the *Iflington* and *German Spa* waters.

BRENT-

BRENTWOOD, *in Essex.*

It is a purging water, of the nature of thofe of Pancras, Epfom, and Dul-wich.

BRISTOL, *in Somerfetfhire.*

The fprings are known by the name of the *Hot Wells.*

The water at its origin is warm, clear, pellucid and fparkling; and if let ftand in a glafs, covers its infide with fmall air-bubbles. It has no fmell, and is foft and agreeable to the tafte. It raifes the thermometer from about feventy to eighty degrees. It contains $12\frac{3}{4}$ grains of chalk, $5\frac{1}{4}$ of muriate of magnefia, and $6\frac{1}{2}$ of fea falt in the gallon.

It has been recommended in a variety of diforders. In confumptions and weaknefs of the lungs; in cafes

H   at-

attended with hectic fever and heat
(in which, among other properties,
it differs from the *Bath* water) in
uterine and other internal hæmorrhages, and in immoderate difcharge of
the menfes; in old diarrhœas and
dyfenteries; in the fluor albus; in
gleets; in the diabetes; and in other
cafes where the fecretions are too
much increafed, and the humours too
thin; in the ftone and gravel; in the
ftrangury; in colliquative fweats;
in fcorbutic and fimilar cafes; in
cholics; in the gout and rheumatifm;
in lofs of appetite and indigeftion; and
in many other difeafes.

The ufual method of drinking the
water is a glafs or two before breakfaft, and about five in the afternoon.
The next day three glaffes before
breakfaft, and as many in the afternoon; and this is to be continued
during the patient's ftay at the Wells.
A quar-

A quarter or half an hour is allowed between each glaſs.

A courſe of theſe waters requires no preparation further than to empty the bowels by ſome gentle purge; and if heat or fever require, to take away a few ounces of blood. Coſtiveneſs, however, ſhould be avoided during the courſe.

Externally they are uſeful in ſore and inflamed eyes; ſcrophulous and cancerous ulcers; and in other ſimilar caſes.

This water is cooling and quenches the thirſt. It is beſt drunk at the ſpring head; though it will bear carriage tolerably well.

BROMLEY, *in Kent.*

It is a chalybeate water, reſembling thoſe of *Spa, Iſlington,* and *Hampſtead.*

BROUGH-

BROUGHTON, *in the Weſt Riding of Yorkſhire, near Coln, in Lancaſhire.*

It is a ſtrong ſulphureous water; it turns ſilver and copper black; it reddens the leaves of trees, &c. and makes the bottom of its baſon black.

It is impregnated with ſea ſalt, and a purging ſalt; and its virtues are ſimilar to thoſe of the *Harrowgate* water.

BUCH, *ſituated about a German mile from the Caroline baths in Bohemia.*

The waters have a briſk pungent taſte, and are plentifully impregnated with *fixed air.* This, on expoſure, flies off, and they become inſipid. In this they differ from *Seltzer* water, which acquires a lixivial taſte by ſtanding.

They contain, however, natron, in the

the proportion of about fixteen grains to the gallon; and therefore their virtues are fimilar to thofe of the *Tilbury* and *Seltzer* waters, but much weaker.

BUGLAWTON, *near Congleton, in Chefhire.*

It is a fulphureous water, impregnated with a purging falt, and in its virtues feems to refemble the *Afkeron* water.

It is intenfely cold, and has a pretty ftrong fulphureous fmell and tafte.

BURLINGTON, *in Yorkfhire.*

It is a brifk chalybeate water, and refembles thofe of *Scarborough* and *Cheltenham,* tho' it feems to be lefs purgative.

BURNLEY, or BOURNLEY, *in Lancafhire.*

It is a chalybeate water of the nature

ture

ture of the *Scarborough,* but lefs purgative.

B u x t o n, *in Derbyfhire.*

This is a hot water, refembling
that of *Briftol.*   It raifes the thermometer to 81° or 82°.

It has a fweet and pleafant tafte.

It contains a little calcareous earth,
together with a fmall quantity of fea
falt, and an inconfiderable portion of
a purging falt.   Iron has been difcovered in it, but in fo extremely fmall
a quantity as not to deferve notice:
and even that perhaps owing to accident.

This water taken inwardly is efteemed good in the diabetes ; in
bloody urine; in the bilious cholic ;
in lofs of appetite, and coldnefs of
the ftomach ; in inward bleedings ;
in atrophy ; in contraction of the
veffels and limbs, efpecially from age;

in

in cramps and convulfions; in the dry afthma without a fever; and alfo in barrennefs.

Inwardly and outwardly it is faid to be good in rheumatic and fcorbutic complaints; in the gout; in inflammation of the liver and kidnies, and in confumptions of the lungs; alfo in old ftrains; in hard callous tumours; in withered and contracted limbs; in the itch, fcabs, nodes, chalky fwellings, ring-worms, and other fimilar complaints.

Befides the hot water, there is alfo a cold *chalybeate* water, with a rough irony tafte. It refembles the *Cáwthorp* water.

CANNOCK, *near Stafford.*

It is one of the beft and lighteft chalybeate waters in Staffordfhire. In its virtues it refembles thofe of *Hampftead* and *Iflington.*

CAPE

CAPE CLEAR, *fituated in the moſt*
ſouthern part of Ireland.

It is a ſmooth, ſaltiſh water, and
lathers with ſoap.

It contains about half a dram of natron, mixed with a little ſea ſalt, in
the gallon.

Its virtues are ſimilar to thoſe of
the waters of *Tilbury* and *Clifton*, but
weaker.

CARGYRLE, *in Wales.*

The ſpring is ſituated about ten or
twelve miles from Cheſter.

The water is of the nature of the
Barrowdale water, but much weaker,
ſeveral quarts being required to be
taken for a purge.

CARLTON, *near Newark upon Trent,*
in the county of Nottingham.

It is chalybeate water, reſembling
thoſe of *Iſlington* and *Hampſtead*, but
it

it has a fœtid fmell, like infufion of horfe-dung.

CAROLINE BATHS, *at Carlfbad, in Bohemia, Germany.*

The waters of this place are hot.

They contain thirty-fix grains of chalk, forty-eight grains of fea falt, one hundred and two grains of natron, and fix drams of vitriolated natron. They are alfo impregnated with iron.

The higheft temperature is 165°, the loweft 114°.

They are recommended externally and internally in female obftructions; in relaxed habits; in glandulous ob-ftructions; in diforders arifing from vifcid fluids, and in a variety of other complaints; and it is faid, that they may be drunk, and bathed in, by per-fons of all ages and conftitutions, with fafety.

CARRICKFERGUS, *in the county of Antrim, Ireland.*

The water is of a blueifh colour, and a very foft tafte, at the fountain-head.

It is weakly purgative; and muft be drank to the quantity of two or three quarts.

Near this fpring is another, a gallon of the water of which affords about an ounce and half of fea falt, and a little vitriolated magnefia, with a quantity of an earthy matter.

CARRICKMORE, *in Ireland.*

It is fituated about five miles from Belturbet, in the county of Cavan.

The water has a foft, milky tafte, like Briftol water; and putrifies by keeping.

It curdles a folution of foap; and with falt of tartar gives a white fediment.

§   It

It contains natron, together with a purging falt.

Its virtues therefore are fimilar to thofe of *Tilbury* and *Clifton.*

CASHMORE, *in the county of Waterford, Ireland.*

It is near the *Crofs-town* water, which it refembles in virtues, though ftronger.

CASTLECONNEL, *in the county of Limerick, Ireland.*

It is a chalybeate water of confiderable repute, and refembles the German *Spa* waters.

CASTLE LOED, *in Rofsfhire, Scotland.*

This is a ftrong fulphureous water. The gallon yielded near $1\frac{4}{5}$ grains of abforbent earth, $26\frac{3}{5}$ of felenite, $30\frac{3}{5}$ of faline matter confifting of vitriolated

H 6   natron

natron with a little fulphur, and probably a fmall portion of marine bittern.

It has been many years in repute
againft cutaneous difeafes.

CASTLEMAIGN, *in the county of
Kerry, Ireland.*

It is a fulphureous, and ftrongly
chalybeate water, and in its virtues
feems to refemble that of *Deddington.*

CAWLEY, *near Dranefield, in Derbyfhire.*

It is fulphureous, and gently purgative; and refembles the *Afkeron*
water.

It contains about half a dram of
vitriolated magnefia in the gallon.

CAWTHORP, *four miles from Bourne,
in Lincolnfhire.*

It is a faltifh chalybeate water, and
foams much as it rifes from the fpring.

It

It refembles the *Tunbridge* water in virtues, but is faid to be more purgative; and is alfo a good corrector of acidities.

CHADLINGTON, *near Chipping-Norton, Oxfordfhire.*

The water has a faltifh tafte, and fmells like the wafhings of a foul gun.

It is one of the waters termed fulphureous.

It contains alfo natron, together with a little fea falt.

It acts as a purgative; and its virtues refemble thofe of the *Sutton Bog* water.

CHAUDE FONTAINE, *about two leagues from Liege, and three from Spa, in Germany.*

The water of thefe fprings is hot, and fupplies fifty baths.

It is claffed by authors with the fulphureous waters; but Dr. Simmons,

mons *, who fpent fome time at this place in 1776 and 1777, informs me they have no fulphureous fmell; that they are impregnated with calcareous earth, and natron, and alfo with fixed air.

They are not chalybeate; and therefore rather refemble our *Briftol* and *Buxton* than the *Bath* water.

Their virtues *externally* however may be collected from what has been faid of the *Aix-la-Chapelle* and *Bath* waters.

CHELTENHAM, *in Glouceferfhire, fix miles from Gloucefter.*

It is one of the beft and moft noted purging chalybeate waters in England, though it is not fo much frequented as formerly.

* The fame gentleman informs me, that on the 5th of July 1777, when the mercury in his thermometer, in the fhade, ftood at 75°, it rofe in the bath to 92°.

The

The gallon contains eight drams of a purging falt, partly vitriolated natron, partly vitriolated magnefia; twenty-five grains of magnefia, part of which is united with marine, part with aerial acid; and nearly five grains of iron combined with aerial acid. It alfo yielded thirty-two ounce meafures of air, twenty-four of which were fixed air, the reft phlogifticated with a portion of hepatic air.

The dofe is from one pint to three or four. It operates with great eafe, and is never attended with gripings, tenefmus, or ftraining at ftool. It is beft taken a little warm.

It alfo creates an appetite; is excellent in fcorbutic complaints, and has been ufed with fuccefs in the gravel.

As the fpring has been calculated to yield only thirty-five pints of water an hour, without frugal management there would not be enough to fupply
the

the demands of the drinkers. The Walton water has lately been recommended as a fubftitute to obviate this inconvenience.

CHIPPENHAM, *in Wiltfhire.*

It is a pretty ftrong chalybeate water, refembling thofe of *Iflington* and *Tunbridge.*

CLEVES, *in the duchy of Cleves, Germany.*

It is a brifk chalybeate water, and operates by urine. It refembles the *Pyrmont* water.

CLIFTON. *This is a village near Deddington, in Oxfordfhire.*

The well is about a furlong fouth of Clifton. The water is clear, and has but little tafte.

The principal ingredient in it is natron, of which about fixty-five grains are contained in the gallon.

Its

Its virtues are fimilar to thofe of the *Tilbury* water, though in a lefs degree. But as it alfo contains a purging falt, it is more purgative than that.

It has been much ufed by way of bath in diforders of the fkin.

COBHAM, *in the county of Surry.*

It is a chalybeate water, of the nature of that of *Tunbridge*, but rather ftronger of the iron.

There is alfo a purging water near it, from a gallon of which Dr. Hals obtained an ounce or upwards of a refiduum, confifting principally of vitriolated magnefia.

CODSALWOOD, *five miles from Wolverhampton, Staffordfhire.*

It is a ftrong fulphureous water.

In its virtues it feems to refemble the *Afkeron* water.

COL-

COLCHESTER, *in the county of Effex.*

It is a purging water of the nature of thofe of *Acton* and *Epfom.*

COLURIAN, *in the parifh of Ludg-van, in Cornwall.*

It is a chalybeate water, and feems to refemble thofe of *Hampftead* and *Iflington.*

COMNER, or CUMNER, *in Berk-fhire, four miles weft of Oxford.*

The water is of a whitifh colour, efpecially in the fummer.

It contains two hundred and forty-four grains of vitriolated magnefia with excefs of the magnefia, and fifty-two of chalk.

It is purgative, and may be drunk to the quantity of one, two, or three

quarts,

quarts, according to the patient's conftitution.

COOLAURAN, *in the county of Fermanagh, Ireland.*

It is a chalybeate water, refembling
that of *Peterhead,* but weaker.

CORSTORPHIN, *two miles from
Edinburgh, Scotland.*

It is a weak fulphureous water,
very flightly impregnated with fea falt,
and vitriolated magnefia.

There is another fpring, about a
mile from Edinburgh, on the banks
of the water of Leith.

They refemble the *Moffat* water in
virtues ; and the latter is reckoned the
ftrongeft.

COVENTRY, *in Warwickſhire.*

It is a chalybeate and purging water,
which fits eafy upon the ftomach,
foon

foon paffes off, raifes the fpirits, and creates an appetite.

In its general virtues it refembles the *Scarborough* and *Cheltenham* waters.

CRICKLE SPA, *fituated near Broughton, in Lancafhire.*

It is a ftrong fulphureous water, a a gallon of which contains about four drams and half of fea falt and vitriolated magnefia, the former of which is greatly predominant, and about fifty grains of calcareous earth.

It is purgative; and in its virtues refembles the *Harrogate* water.

About a mile diftant is Broughton water, of the fame nature, but containing lefs fea falt.

CROFT, *in the North Riding of Yorkfhire, on the confines of Durham.*

This is a ftrong fulphureous water, a gallon of which contains one hundred
dred

dred and fifty grains of calcareous earth, thirty of vitriolated magnefia, and ten of fea falt.

It is clear and fparkling, and its ftream does not rife or fall by rain or drought.

It is purgative, and of the nature of the *Afkeron* water; and is faid to have performed remarkable cures.

CROSS-TOWN, *near the town of Waterford, Ireland.*

It refembles the *Hartfell* water in Scotland.

This water vomits fome, purges others, and with others operates by urine.

It feems at fome times to contain a greater quantity of acid than at others.

CUNLEY-HOUSE, *near Whaley, in Lancafhire.*

It is ftrongly fulphureous, and gently

ly purgative, and feems to refemble
in its virtues the *Afkeron* water.

D A s W I L D - B A D, *within the walls
of the town of Nuremberg, Germany.*

It is a chalybeate water, with a fub-
aftringent tafte, and contains alfo a
faline matter.

It has been recommended in obftructions of the vifcera, and in female
complaints.

D' A x e n F o i x, *about fifteen leagues
weft of Thouloufe, France.*

This place abounds with hot fulphureous waters of different temperatures. They are recommended as
baths, or otherwife, in thofe complaints in which the *Aix-la-Chapelle*
and *Barèges* waters are ferviceable.

D E D D I N G T O N.

This is a fulphureous chalybeate
water;

water; but foon lofes its fulphureous fmell by keeping.

Drunk in large quantities it is purgative; and in lefs dofes as an alterative, it is good in fcorbutic and cutaneous diforders.

DERBY, *near to the town of Derby, in Derbyfhire.*

It is a chalybeate water of the nature of that of *Tunbridge,* but feems to be ftronger.

DERRINDAFF, *in the county of Cavan, Ireland.*

This is a fulphureous water, impregnated with a purging falt.

Its virtues refemble thofe of the *Afkeron* water.

DERRYHENCE, or DERRYINCH, *in the county of Fermanagh, Ireland.*

The water is fulphureous.

It

It alfo contains natron, and refembles in its virtues the waters of *Drumgoon* and *Swadlingbar*.

D E R R Y L E S T E R, *in the county of Cavan, about three miles from Swadlingbar, Ireland.*

The water is of the nature of that of Drumgoon, but contains much lefs of the falts.

D O G A N D D U C K.

A noted tea-drinking houfe in St. George's Fields, near London; and in the fpring and fummer months the waters are much reforted to.

The water is clear, and has but little tafte.

It is a mild purgative, containing vitriolated magnefia mixed with fea falt, and may be drank to the quantity of feveral pints. Moft frequently, however, it is quickened by the
addition

addition of Glauber's, or other purging falts.

It is of ufe in fcrophulous complaints, leprofies and difeafes of the fkin ; and is alfo faid to prevent the return of cancerous difeafes. For thefe complaints it may be ufed both internally and externally.

It is cooling and diuretic ; and may be given freely to young people of robuft conftitutions. But it cools and relaxes people in years and of weak habits too much. It is alfo apt to bring on or increafe the fluor albus in weakly women.

DORTSHILL, *near Litchfield, in Staffordfhire.*

The water is a brifk chalybeate, fimilar to that of *Tunbridge.*

There is alfo a faline purging water of the nature of the *Barrowdale* water, but much weaker.

I   DRI-

DRIBURG, *about half a mile from the town of Driburg, in Weſtphalia.*

The water, which is in the higheſt reputation abroad, very much reſembles the *Pyrmont*; containing the ſame ingredients, but in a rather larger proportion.

The quantity of fixed air obtained from it by Dr. Higgins was to that of Pyrmont as thirteen to twelve.

DRIG WELL, *near Revenglas, in Cumberland.*

This is a briſk, ſpirituous, ſulphureous chalybeate; and in its virtues reſembles the *Deddington* water.

DROPPING WELL, *at Knareſborough, in Yorkſhire.*

It is very cold, limpid, and ſweettaſted; and in time petrifies ſubſtances thrown into it.

In

In its virtues it refembles the *New-ton Dale* water. The dofe has formerly been feveral quarts in a day; but three or four half pints are now judged fufficient.

Its ufe fhould be preceded by a dofe or two of rhubarb.

DRUMASNAVE, *called likewife Mount Campbell, in the County of Leitrim, Ireland.*

This is one of the ftrongeft ful-phureous waters in Ireland, as is fhewn by its quick and ftrong effect in difcolouring metals.

It is perfectly clear and limpid in common; but before rain becomes white.

It contains about twelve grains of natron, with a fmall quantity of purging falt, in the gallon.

It operates powerfully by urine,

and

and purges fome conftitutions, but is
faid to render others coftive.

DRUMGOON, *in the county of Fermanagh, Ireland.*

The water has a ftrong fulphureous
fmell, and tinges filver of a copper
colour in a few minutes. It alfo depofits a black fediment at the bottom
of the well.

It contains near a dram of natron
in the gallon, with a little fea falt.

It is recommended for the cure of
cutaneous and fcrophulous diforders;
and for worms.

There are two other fulphureous
fprings in the neighbourhood; the
one nearly refembles this; the other
is more of a purgative nature.

DUB

DUBLIN SALT SPRINGS. *There are five of these Springs in* Francis Street, *and one in* Thomas's Court.

The waters are falt, and of the nature of *Barrowdale* water. For a purge, they muft be taken to the quantity of feveral pints. They operate without griping.

DULWICH. *The Spring is fituated between Dulwich and Lewisham, in the county of Kent.*

The water is clear, and has a brackifh tafte, leaving a bitternefs in the throat.

It contains a purging falt, together with fea falt.

This is a celebrated purging water; is alfo diuretic; and is recommended in a variety of diforders.

It is particularly of ufe in complaints arifing from obftructions; as

I 3 thofe

thofe of the liver, fpleen, and other vifcera.

It is recommended in the green ficknefs, the jaundice, the fcurvy, in difficulty of urine, and in gravelly complaints.

It is faid to ftrengthen the ftomach, and create a good digeftion.

It is alfo faid to ftrengthen the nervous fyftem, and therefore to be ferviceable in palfies, apoplexies, and other nervous diforders. In thefe cafes it is beft taken warm.

The courfe of drinking this water is ufually twenty days. Three pints a day are to be drunk at firft; it fhould be increafed to eight pints by the tenth day, and afterwards decreafed in the fame manner.

A new fpring has fince been difcovered, whofe virtues are fimilar to thofe of the old one, but it is ftronger.

DUN-

DUNNARD, *about eighteen miles from Dublin.*
This is a chalybeate water, refembling that of *Peterhead*, but weaker.

DUNSE, *in Scotland.*
It is a chalybeate water, fimilar to that of *Tunbridge*.

DURHAM. *The Spring is fituated near Durham, on the north fide of the river Ware.*
It is a ftrong fulphureous water, and is alfo impregnated with fea falt, of which it contains thirty-eight grains in the gallon.

In its virtues it refembles the *Harrogate* water.

Near to this, in the middle of the river, is a falt fpring, which is drunk as a purging water.

EGRA, *in Bohemia.*
This is a fpirity chalybeate water,

I 4   and

and operates both by ſtool and urine.
It contains leſs fixed air than the *Pyrmont* water, but is more purgative.
It abounds with vitriolated magneſia
mixed with muriate of magneſia.

ENGHIEN, or ANGUIEN, *a city of Hainault.*

This water contains ſulphur, vitriolated magneſia, chalk, and magneſia.

EPSOM, *in Surry, about ſixteen miles from London.*

The water has a ſlight ſaline taſte,
is clear, and without ſmell.   But if
it be kept in covered veſſels for ſome
weeks in the ſummer it will ſtink,
and acquire a nauſeous and ſaltiſh
bitter taſte.

This was the firſt water from which
the bitter purging ſalt (thence called
Epſom ſalt) was obtained.   But the
ſalt

falt ufually fold by that name is different from that yielded by the Epfom water, though perhaps not inferior in virtue. It is made from the bittern left after the chryftallization of common falt from fea water.

The Epfom water is purgative; for which purpofe it muft be drank to the quantity of two or three pints. It alfo operates by urine.

Taken in lefs quantity (about the third part of a pint three times a day) it is a mild alterative, and good in thofe complaints for which the *Acton* and *Pancras* waters are recommended.

It is likewife efteemed good for wafhing old fores.

FAIRBURN, *in the county of Rofs, in Scotland.*

This is about two miles from the

Caftle-

Caftle-Loed well, which it nearly refembles, but is fomewhat weaker.

FELSTEAD, *in Eſſex.*

The fpring is fituated at the bottom
of a rock. The water is a light chalybeate, refembling that of *Iſlington.*

FILAH, *near Scarborough, in York-
ſhire.*

This is a falt chalybeate water, and
is ufed by the common people as a
purgative; for which purpofe they
drink to the quantity of feveral quarts:
it alfo operates by urine.

FRANKFORT, *in Germany.*

There are two ftrong fulphureous
waters in the neighbourhood of Frank-
fort on the Maine.

The one is called FAULPUMP,

The

The other FONS SCABIOSORUM.

They are alſo impregnated with ſea ſalt, and are of the nature of the *Moffat* and *Harrogate* waters.

GAINSBOROUGH, *in Lincolnſhire.*

This is a weak ſulphureous chalybeate water, ſimilar to that of *Deddington.*

GALWAY, *in the county of Galway, Ireland.*

It is a chalybeate water, of the nature of that of *Tunbridge.*

GLANMILE, *near Naul, in Ireland.*

It is a chalybeate water, reſembling that of *Peterhead,* but weaker.

GLASTONBURY, *in Somerſetſhire.*

This water is of the ſame nature

I 6   with

with thofe of *Tilbury* and *Clifton*;
but weaker than either of thefe.

It has alfo a fmall mixture of fea
falt.

It is naturally fweet, but by keeping becomes putrid.

This water was formerly in great
repute; and many fuperftitions were
held concerning it; but it has not
lately been efteemed.

GLENDY, *in the county of Mairns,
Scotland.*

This is a ftrong chalybeate water,
little inferior to that of *Peterhead.*

GRANSHAW, *near Dunnaghadee,
in the county of Down, Ireland.*

It is a chalybeate water, of the nature of that of *Caftle Connel.*

GROS-

GROSSENENDORF, *about five leagues from Hanover.*

This is a cold fulphureous water, of fome repute in the gout, palfy, and difeafes of the fkin and breaft.

The Landgrave of Heffe Caffel, in whofe dominions it is, has lately directed baths and other conveniences to be built here for the accommodation of invalids.

GUGGA.

See *Kuka.*

HAIGH, *near Wigan, in Lancashire.*

It is impregnated with green vitriol; and is of the nature of the *Shadwell* water; which fee.

It works plentifully by vomit, and ftool; and is excellent for ftopping inward bleeding.

HAMP-

HAMPSTEAD.

This is a chalybeate water, of the nature of that of *Iflington*, but fomewhat ftronger. The dofe is from half a pint to feveral pints.

It was formerly, and perhaps defervedly, in great repute.

This water is better in the morning than in the middle of the day; and in cold weather it is much ftronger than in hot.

HANBRIDGE, *in Lancaſhire*.

It is a chalybeate water, of the nature of that of *Scarborough*, but lefs purgative.

HANLYS, *near Shrewſbury, in Shrop-ſhire*.

The water is clear, and limpid, and has a faline and bitter, though not difagreeable tafte.

It fprings up with impetuofity at
the

the fountain; and does not change colour, or lofe its virtue, by being expofed to the air.

It is purgative; and the dofe is from two to four half pints.

The gallon yields one hundred and twenty grains of vitriolated magnefia.

At this place there is alfo a *chalybeate water.* It is near to the purging water, and is of the nature of thofe of *Scarborough* and *Landrindod.*

It is brifk and pungent to the tafte, and as it is taken from the fountain, clear, and not unpleafant; but lofes its virtues by keeping.

HARROGATE, *near Knarefborough, Yorkfhire.*

There are four fprings at this place, but the waters of all of them are nearly alike, except in the quantity of the faline matter they contain.

Of

Of the three old fprings, the higheft gave three ounces of folid matter ; the loweft, an ounce and half ; and the middle one, only half an ounce. Of the latter one hundred and forty grains were earth.

The water as it fprings up is clear and fparkling, and throws up a quantity of air-bubbles.

It has a ftrong fmell of fulphur, and is fuppofed to be the ftrongeft fulphureous water in England.

It has a falt tafte, as it contains a confiderable quantity of fea falt, together with a little marine falt of magnefia, and calcareous earth.

It is purgative ; and the dofe required for this purpofe is about three or four pints.

When drank in fmaller quantities, it is a good alterative, and is found ferviceable in the fcurvy, king's evil, and difeafes of the fkin. It may be ufed

uſed at the ſame time outwardly, by
way of bath, or fomentation.

It has been found efficacious in de-
ſtroying worms.

It has been recommended in the
gout, jaundice, the ſpleen, the green
ſickneſs, and other diſorders ariſing
from obſtructions.

It is uſed externally for removing
old aches, ſtrains, paralytic weakneſſes,
and the like. Alſo for the cure of
ulcers, ſcabs, the itch, &c.

N. B. Between *Harrogate* and *Knareſ-*
borough, are alſo ſeveral *chalyb-*
eate waters, which ſeem to reſemble thoſe of *Hampſtead* and *Iſling-*
ton. The moſt remarkable are,
the *Allum Well*, the *Sweet Spa*, and
the *Tuewhet Well*. The latter is
the ſtrongeſt.

HART-

HARTFELL, *in the county of An-nandale, Scotland.*

It is impregnated with green vi-triol, and refembles the *Shadwell* wa-ter, but is much weaker.

It is recommended in inward bleed-ings, in immoderate flux of the men-fes, in dyfenteries, in bloody urine, in the fluor albus, in gleets, in com-plaints of the ftomach and bowels, and in confumptions.

The dofe is from a gill to a pint or two, taken at repeated draughts in the morning.

Externally, it cures itchy, and tet-terous eruptions, and old fores, efpe-cially if taken at the fame time as an internal remedy.

HARTLEPOOL, *in Durham.*

This is a fine clear chalybeate wa-ter ;

ter; with a flight fulphureous fmell, and pleafant tafte.

It is alfo diuretic and laxative; and is recommended as excellent in fcorbutic complaints, in bilious and nervous cholics, in pains of the ftomach and indigeftion, in the gravel, in female obftructions, in the hypochondriacal difeafe, in cachexy, in hectical heats, and in recent ulcers.

HOLT, *near Bradford, in Wiltfhire.*

The water is limpid, and has but little tafte.

It contains a purging falt, together with a large quantity of earth.

On account of the latter ingredient, it is but a very mild purge, and two quarts are ufually required to produce any confiderable operation this way.

Taken in lefs quantity it is alterative, and diuretic.

It is alfo good as a diluent, cooler, and

and ſtrengthener; and creates an appetite.

Externally, rags, or ſpunge dipt in it, are ſaid to cure ſcrophulous ulcers, attended with carious bones; an internal courſe being obſerved at the ſame time.

It is alſo of ſervice in old running ulcers of the legs, and other parts; in cutaneous foulneſſes, tho' attehded with hot corroſive humours; in the piles, in cancerous ulcers, and in foreneſſes of the eyes. But in theſe caſes alſo it muſt be uſed both internally and externally.

Hol t, *near Market-Harborough, in Leiceſterſhire.*
See *Nevil-Holt.*

Jessop's Well, *on Stoke Common, near Cobham, in Surry.*

This is a ſtrong purging water, with

with a naufeous tafte, and is alfo
flightly chalybeate.

Drank to about a quart, it purges
brifkly without griping, and operates
likewife by urine.

It alfo enlivens the fpirits, and as
the dofe is fmaller than that of other
purging waters, it fits better on the
ftomach.

It lofes its virtues by being kept.

Taken in lefs dofes as an alterative,
it is a good antifcorbutic.

ILMINGTON, *in Warwickfhire, on
the borders of Worcefterfhire.*

This a very clear and fparkling
chalybeate water, abounding in fixed
air, and impregnated alfo with natron.

It preferves its virtues for feveral
weeks in bottles well corked; though
if expofed to the air, it lofes them in
twenty-four hours.

It

It operates by urine; and it alſo ſometimes purges.

It is recommended as excellent in ſcorbutic complaints, in obſtructions of the liver and ſpleen, in the jaundice, in beginning dropſies, in the gravel, and obſtruction of urine, and in diſorders ariſing from acidity.

Externally, it is good for old running ſores, ſcorbutic eruptions, and the like.

INGLEWHITE, *in Lancaſhire*.

It is a ſtrong chalybeate ſulphureous water, and is good in ſcorbutic, and cutaneous diſeaſes. But it will not purge unleſs Glauber's, or ſome other ſalt be added to it.

ISLINGTON, *in the county of Middleſex, near London*.

This is a ſlight chalybeate water, ſtriking

ftriking a purple or blackifh colour with galls, and is reckoned one of the beft of the kind about London.

The iron in this water is held in folution by means of *fixed air*, or *aërial acid*, as in the Pyrmont water. If, after the fixed air has efcaped, and the iron (which it held in folution) precipitates, the water be left to pu‑ trify, the fixed air difengaged by the putrefaction again diffolves the iron, and caufes it to be fufpended in the water; it then recovers its chalybeate tafte, and property of tinging black with galls, both which it had loft before.

It is recommended in indigeftion, and lofs of appetite, in lownefs of fpirits, nervous, hyfteric, and hypo‑ chondriacal complaints, and relaxed conftitutions, and raifes the fpirits greatly. It is good in the fluor albus, in weakneffes from mifcarriage, in obftructions of the liver, the kidnies, &c.

&c. It is alfo ferviceable in difeafes of the fkin, in fcorbutic complaints, in the gravel, and in paralytic diforders.

It operates chiefly by urine, and may be drunk to the quantity of feveral half pints, or even pints, according to the patient's conftitution.

This water was formerly in great repute, and deferves to be more frequented than it is at prefent.

KANTURK, *in-the county of Cork, Ireland.*

It is a chalybeate water, of the nature of that of *Peterhead,* but weaker.

KEDDLESTONE, *in Derbyfhire.*

This is a ftrong fulphureous water, and ftinks intolerably.

It is extremely clear at the fountain, but by ftanding becomes blackifh. It prefently

prefently turns filver of a black copper colour.

It contains thirty-eight grains of
fea falt, and forty-two grains of calcareous earth in a gallon.

Its virtues refemble thofe of the
Harrogate water.

KENSINGTON, *in the county of*
Middlefex, near London.

It is a purging water, of the nature of thofe of *Acton* and *Pancras.*

KILBREW, *in the county of Meath,*
Ireland.

This is a ftrong vitriolic chalybeate
water, and refembles the *Shadwell*
water.

Half a pint vomits and purges.

When taken as an alterative it
fhould be ufed with great caution,
beginning with a fmall quantity, and
increafing the dofe.

K   It

It is recommended in the fluor albus, in immoderate fluxes from the womb, in obftinate intermittents, and in dropfies.

KILBURN, *in Middlefex, near London.*

It is a purging water, like thofe of *Bagnigge Wells, Dulwich,* &c.

KILLINGSHANVALLY, *in the county of Fermanagh, Ireland.*

This is a chalybeate water, and is alfo diuretic and gently laxative. It feems to refemble the *Hanlys* chalybeate water.

KILLASHER, *in the county of Fermanagh, Ireland.*

The water is ftrongly fulphureous, and contains natron.

Its virtues refemble thofe of the *Swadlingbar* water.

KIL-

KILROOT, *in the county of Antrim,*
Ireland.

It is of the nature of *Barrowdale*
water, but weaker; several pints being
required for a purge.

KINALTON, or KYNOLTON, *a*
village in Nottinghamſhire.

The water is limpid and cooling,
with a ſomewhat ſaltiſh taſte.

It is purging; but is weaker than
the Epſom water, and therefore muſt
be drunk plentifully.

A gallon contains about one hundred and fifty grains only of vitriolated magneſia.

KINCARDINE, *in the county of*
Mairns, Scotland.

This is a chalybeate water, little
inferior in ſtrength to that of *Peter-*
head.

KINGSCLIFF, *in Northamptonſhire.*

It is a chalybeate laxative water, and reſembles the *Scarborough* and *Cheltenham* waters.

KIRBY, or KIRKBY-THOWER, *in Weſtmoreland.*

There are two ſprings nearly of the ſame kind, only the lower one is reckoned the ſtrongeſt chalybeate.

The water of both is clear, fine, and has a chalybeate ſweetiſh taſte. Drunk to the quantity of ſeveral quarts it is purgative.   It is alſo a good corrector of acidities.

KNARESBOROUGH.

See *Dropping Well.*

KNOWSLEY, *in Lancaſhire.*

This is a ſlight acidulous chalybeate water, and both taſtes and ſmells of iron.

If

If drunk to four or five pints it is laxative.

It refembles the *Scarborough* and *Cheltenham* waters in virtue, though it feems to be lefs purgative.

KORYTNA, *near Hunnobroda, in Moravia, Germany.*

It is fituated on a high and almoft inacceffible rock, in the midft of a thick wood.

It has a very fœtid difagreeable tafte, and a black colour; and there is much mud at the bottom of the well.

It is reckoned the ftrongeft fulphu‑reous water in that country.

KUKA, *in the county of Graditz, in Bohemia, near the town of Jaro‑mitz, at the conflux of the rivers Elbe and Orlitz, Germany.*

This is a very brifk chalybeate wa‑

K 3   ter,

ter, highly impregnated with fixed air, and alfo with natron. It has a grateful and fomewhat pleafant tafte, and a pungent fmell, which affects the whole head. If it be heated, it emits a penetrating acid fulphureous fmelling vapour. It will not bear carriage.

It operates chiefly by infenfible perfpiration ; and fometimes by fpitting, by fweat, and by urine.

In its general virtues it refembles the *German Spa* waters.

LA MARQUISE, et LA MARIE.
See *Vahls*.

LANCASTER, or SALE'S SP
in Lancafhire.

This is a clear chalybeate water, powerfully diuretic, gently purgative, and vomits if taken to the quantity of feveral quarts.

Taken

'Taken as an alternative it has the general virtues of the *Tunbridge* water.

LATHAM, *in Lancashire.*

It is a fine chryftalline chalybeate, of the nature of the *Tunbridge* water.

LLANDRINDOD, *in the county of Radnor, South Wales.*

In this place there are three mineral fprings :

1ft. *The faline pump,* or *purging water.*

2d. *The fulphureous water,* commonly called *the black ftinking well.*

3. *The chalybeate rock water.*

The faline purging, or *pump water,* may be ufed as a *purge* twice in a week. It is directed to be drunk at the fountain-head by half pints, till it begins to operate; the patient walking or riding about between each draught. It operates alfo by urine.

For an *alterative,* about three pints
are directed to be drunk in a day.   A
pint and half in the morning before
breakfaſt, at three draughts, a quarter of an hour between each half
pint.   The other pint and half likewiſe at three draughts : one an hour
before dinner; another about ſix
o'clock in the evening; and the third
going to bed.   If the body remain
coſtive, the quantity muſt be increaſ-
ed.   The courſe ſhould be continued
ſeveral weeks; and the moſt proper
ſeaſon is the ſummer.

It is alſo uſed as a bath and fomentation.

It is recommended both internally
and externally in the ſcurvy, leproſy,
tetters, King's evil, and all cutaneous
foulneſſes.

It is alſo preſcribed in the gravel,
the hypochondriacal diſeaſe, indigeſtion, and in other complaints.

The

The fulphureous water; called alfo *the black ftinking water,* from its ftrong fmell, and the blacknefs of the channel through which it paffes.

The quantity to be drunk cannot in general be determined: but it is beft to begin with fmall dofes, from a pint to a quart in the morning, taken at repeated draughts. The quantity may be increafed as the conftitution will bear; or as much as will fit eafy on the ftomach, and pafs off well. When it gives the leaft uneafinefs, it is a fign that the dofe is too large.

It is alfo ufed outwardly, by way of bath or fomentation.

It is recommended in a variety of complaints. In the King's evil, fcurvy, leprofy, and all cutaneous dif-eafes; in the jaundice, hypochon-driacal, and other diforders arifing from obftruction; in the gravel, rheu-matifm, gout, bloody flux, hectic

fever,

fever, weakneffes of the limbs, want of digeftion, and many others.

The chalybeate, or *rock water,* is limpid and tranfparent, as taken from the fountain, but on ftanding foon lofes thefe qualities, together with its chalybeate tafte. Mixed with fugar and rough cyder as it is taken up from the fpring, it excites a brifk fermentation.

It is recommended in fuch chronic diftempers as proceed from laxity of the fibres, and weaknefs of the mufcular fyftem; in weaknefs of the nerves; in paralytic complaints; and the like.

It is alfo good in fcorbutic cafes; in moift and convulfive afthmas; in obftinate agues; in obftructions of the lower belly; in wandering, flow, nervous fevers; and in diforders arifing from obftruction.

LLANGYBI, *in Caernarvonshire,*
North Wales.

The water has a harsh taste, in-
clining to bitter.

It has been found efficacious in
diforders of the eyes; in the King's
evil; fcald heads; ulcers; eruptions
of the skin; the fcurvy; the itch, &c.
Alfo in rheumatisms, palfy, and con-
vulfion fits.

This water has long been in repute
in the neighbourhood.

LEAMINGTON.

This is of the nature of *Barrow-*
dale water, but much weaker, containing little more than a fourth of the
fame ingredients in an equal quantity.
The dofe for a purge is from a quart
to four or five pints, and it likewife
ufually vomits.

K 6   LEEZ,

LEEZ, *near the Earl of Manchefter's,
Effex.*

It is a chalybeate water, fimilar to
thofe of *Iflington* and *Hampftead*.

LINCOMB, *near Bath, in Somerfetfhire.*

This is a chalybeate and acidulous
water, containing natron, with a fmall
quantity of purging falt.   It foon
lofes its virtue if expofed to the air;
and in a few days alfo in bottles.

It refembles, in its virtues, the waters of *Thetford* and *Ilmington*.

LISBEAK, *in the parifh of Killafher,
in the county of Fermanagh, Ireland.*

Here are two ftrong fulphureous
waters, much of the fame kind.

They yield upwards of thirty grains
of natron in the gallon, and it is more

free

free from heterogeneous mixtures than
in moſt waters.

LIS-DONE-VARNA, *in the county of Clare, in Ireland.*

This is a ſtrong chalybeate water,
and manifeſts itſelf as ſuch both to the
taſte and ſmell. It is alſo impregnated
with natron.

It keeps its virtue in well-corked
bottles.

It uſually vomits and purges on firſt
drinking, but afterwards operates by
urine.

It ſeems to reſemble, in virtues,
the *Thetford* and *Ilmington* waters.

LOANSBURY, *in Lord Burlington's park, in Yorkſhire.*

This is a ſulphureous water, weakly
impregnated with a purging ſalt.

It ſeems to be of the nature of the
Alkeron water; but is only uſed at preſent

fent for wafhing mangy dogs and fcabby horfes.

MACCROOMP, *in Ireland, about fix-teen miles from Cork.*

This is a chalybeate water, impregnated with natron, and refembles the *Thetford* and *Ilmington* waters.

MAHEREBERG, *fituated near Branden Bay, in the county of Kerry, Ireland.*

It is of the nature of the *Barrowdale* water, but contains a much fmaller quantity of fea falt. The dofe for a purge is from a pint to a quart.

MALLOW, *in the county of Cork, Ireland.*

This is a warm water, perfe&ly limpid and pleafant-tafted, and keeps long in bottles well corked.

It

It is recommended in moſt caſes for which the *Briſtol* water has been uſed.

MALTON. *The Spring lies at the weſt end of the town of New Malton, in Yorkſhire.*

It is a ſtrong chalybeate, abounding with fixed air when freſh drawn; has a ſaltiſh taſte, and leaves a bitterneſs in the throat.

A gallon yields nearly two drams of vitriolated magneſia.

It operates by ſtool and urine. The doſe is from three pints to twice that quantity. If the ſtomach be foul, it is apt to vomit. In its virtues it reſembles the *Scarborough* water.

MALVERN, *in Glouceſterſhire.*

There are two noted ſprings at this place, one of them called the *Holy Well,* in the midway between Great and Little Malvern, the other is about

a quara quarter of a mile from Great Malvern. But the waters are not materially different.

They are light and pleafant chalybeates, and are remarkable for being almoft entirely free from any earthy matter; for three quarts of the Holy Well water being evaporated, fcarce the fourth part of a grain of fediment was left behind.

They are recommended as excellent in difeafes of the fkin; leprofies; fcorbutic complaints; the King's evil; glandular obftrudions; fcald heads; old fores; cancers, &c. They are alfo ferviceable in inflammations and other difeafes of the eyes; in the gout and ftone; in cachedic, bilious, and paralytic cafes; in old head-achs, and in female obftrudions.

The external ufe is by wafhing the part under the fpout feveral times in a day; afterwards covering the part with cloths

cloths dipt in the water, which muſt be kept conſtantly moiſt. Thoſe who bathe, uſually go into the water with their linen on, and dreſs upon it wet, and it is never found to be attended with inconvenience.

The waters, when firſt drunk, are apt to occaſion, in ſome, a ſlight nauſea; others they purge briſkly for ſeveral days; but they operate by urine in all.

It is adviſeable to drink freely of the waters for ſome days before they are uſed externally.

MARKSHALL, *in Eſſex.*

This is a chalybeate water, reſembling thoſe of *Iſlington* and *Hampſtead.*

MATLOCK, *near Wirkſworth, in Derbyſhire.*

At this place (which is perfectly romantic) are ſeveral ſprings of warm water,

water, which appear to be of the nature of the *Bristol* water, except that
it is very slightly impregnated with
iron.

Its heat is about 69°, and its virtues
are similar to those of the *Bristol* and
Buxton waters.

The baths are recommended in
rheumatic complaints, in cutaneous
disorders, and in other cases where
warm bathing is serviceable.

There are great numbers of petri-
factions in the course of this water.

MAUDSLEY, *near Preston, in Lancashire.*

The water is of a blueish colour,
has a fœtid smell, and a brackish taste.

It is a strong sulphureous water,
and contains about two ounces of sea
salt in the gallon.

It is purgative, and has nearly the
same virtues as the *Harrogate* water.

MECHAN,

MECHAN, *in the county of Fermanagh, Ireland.*

In this place there are two fulphureous fprings, both of the fame nature.

They contain natron, and in their virtues refemble the *Drumgoon* and *Swadlingbar* waters.

MILLAR's SPA, *Stockport, in the county of Lancafter,*

It is a chalybeate water of the nature of that of *Tunbridge,* but feems to be ftronger of the iron.

MOFFAT, *in the county of Annandale, Scotland.*

At this place there are two fprings or wells.

They are both fulphureous, and have a ftrong fmell and tafte; the upper one is the ftrongeft, and moft naufeous, and lefs drunk of than the other, though as it bears heat better it is moft ufed for bathing.

The

The Moffat water is alterative, and diuretic, but it fometimes purges.

From a gallon were obtained three grains of earth, and fifty grains of marine falt, though probably mixed with a fmall quantity of vitriolated magnefia.

It being fufpected by Dr. Plummer to contain copper, the Rev. D . Walker put a polifhed plate of iron into the well, and he found after fome time it had contracted a green ruft. This, in his opinion, confirms Dr. Plummer's conjecture.

MORETON, or MORETON-SEE, *fituated about two miles weft of Market-Drayton, in Shropfhire.*

It is efteemed as an excellent cooling and diuretic purge. It operates brifkly ; is pungent to the tafte, and feems to be of the nature of *Holt* water.

The gallon contains 200 grains of
vitri-

vitriolated magnefia, and 76 of calcareous earth.

MOSS HOUSE, *near Maudſley, in Lancaſhire.*

This is a briſk chalybeate water,
and in its virtues refembles thofe of
Hampſtead and *Iſlington.*

MOUNT D'OR, *ſeven leagues from Clermont, in the Auvergne, France.*

The water is warm, and of the nature of the *Aix-la-Chapelle.*

Taken internally it acts as a diuretic, and it fometimes purges. Bathing
in it fweats profufely, without weak-
ening the patient.

It has been recommended in the
rheumatifm, gout, palfy, and many
other diforders.

MOUNT PALLAS, *in the county of Cavan, Ireland.*

It is a chalybeate water, and feems
to be of the nature of the *Athlone.*

NEVIL-

N E V I L - H O L T, *near Market-*
Harborough, in Leicefterfhire.

This is an exceeding clear water as
it falls from the fpout, and is void of
all fmell. It has a brifk, auftere, bitter, yet not difagreeable, tafte, and
abounds in fixed air.

Expofed to the air, it foon becomes
turbid, and fpoils. But in well-clofed
bottles it will keep good.

A gallon of the water contains two
drams of vitriolated magnefia, two
drams eighteen grains of muriated argillaceous earth, and eighteen grains
of muriated magnefia.

Drunk to the quantity of feveral
pints, it proves purgative, and operates without griping.

It alfo operates by urine and fweat.

It is a powerful antifeptic in putrid difeafes.

When taken as an alterative, it muft
be

be taken in small doses, from a few spoonfuls to a quarter or half a pint, several times in a day, according to its effect; and a little brandy, or the like, may be added if it sit cold on the stomach.

It is esteemed an excellent remedy in old dysenteries and diarrhœas, in internal hæmorrhages, in the fluor albus, and gleets, in the gravel, in rheumatisms, and for the worms; it is good in atrophies, in bloated constitutions, and dropsical complaints, in scorbutic disorders, in want of appetite, and in other cases; in inflammatory complaints however, and where there is an acidity of the humours, it does mischief.

Externally, it is a speedy cure for fresh wounds, for inflamed eyes, and hectic ulcers, &c. especially if taken inwardly at the same time.

NEW

8

New Cartmal.

See *Rougham*.

Newnham Regis, *in Warwick-shire.*

There are three wells at this place: they are all of them chalybeate, laxative, and diuretic; and feem to refemble the *Scarborough* water.

They have fomewhat of a fulphureous fmell.

Newton Dale, *in the North Riding of Yorkfhire.*

This is a cold petrifying water.

It is faid to cure effectually loofeneffes, and bleedings of every kind; and that it reftore's weakened joints, though beginning to be diftorted, by bathing in it.

New-

NEWTON STEWART, *near Caf-
tlebill, in the county of Tyrone, Ireland.*

It is a chalybeate water, of the nature of that of *Tunbridge.*

NEZDENICE, *in Germany, about
half a mile from Hunnobroda, in the
diſtriEt of the caſtle of Banow. The
Spring is near this village.*

This is an acidulous water, impregnated with fixed air like thoſe of *Seltzer* and *Pyrmont.*

It is in great repute among the people in the neighbourhood, for the cure
of many diſorders, particularly thoſe
in which the waters juſt mentioned
are ſerviceable.

NOBBER, *in the county of Meath,
Ireland.*

It is a vitriolic water, and reſembles thoſe of *Hartfell* and *Croſs-town.*

L   NOR-

NORMANBY, *four miles from Pick-
ering, in Yorkſhire.*

It is clear, beautiful, and fœtid,
and when poured out ſparkles like
Champagne.

It is a ſulphureous, and gently purgative water, and reſembles the *Aſkeron* water in virtues. A gallon yields
ſcarcely twenty grains of vitriolated
magneſia, and about half that quantity of ſea ſalt.

Near it is a chalybeate water, called *Nether Normanby Spa*; a gallon of
which afforded ten grains of ſea ſalt.

NORTH-HALL.
See *Barnet.*

NOTTINGTON, *near Weymouth,
in Dorſetſhire.*

This is a ſtrong ſulphureous water.

Its flavour reſembles that of boiled
eggs; and its colour, in a tin veſſel,
is

is blue. A fhilling put into it at the fountain-head, becomes, in a few minutes, blue.

It contains 30 grains of natron, and feven of earth, in the gallon.

It is in repute for curing foulneffes of the fkin.

ORSTON, *in the county of Notting-ham, near Thoroton.*

This water has a delicious, gentle, rough, fweetifh, chalybeate tafte, and a flight fulphureous fmell. It is replete with fixed air, fparkles and flies when poured out into a glafs, and makes the heads of thofe who drink it giddy.

It foon fpoils by expofure to air.

It is purgative, and feems to be poffeffed of the fame virtues as the *Pyrmont* water, for which it may be ufed as a fubftitute.

OUL-

O U L T O N, *in Norfolk.*

It is a flight chalybeate water, fimilar to that of *Iflington.*

O W E N   B R E U N, *in the county of Cavan, Ireland.*

This is a fulphureous water, impregnated with a purging falt, and a little natron.

Its virtues refemble thofe of the *Afkeron* water.

P A N C R A S, *in Middlefex, near London.*

The water is almoft infipid to the tafte.

It is impregnated with a purging falt, together with a fmall portion of fea falt.

It is therefore a purgative water, and is alfo diuretic.

Its

Its virtues are allied to thofe of the *Cheltenham* water, and it is alfo of fervice in the ftone, gravel, and fimilar diforders.

PASSY, *near Paris, in France.*

It is a clear, colourlefs, chalybeate water, with a fubacid tafte, and ferruginous fmell, and emits plenty of air-bubbles.

It is a ftrong chalybeate water, but does not prove purgative, unlefs drunk in large quantity. It is of the nature of *Pyrmont* water.

PETERHEAD, *in the county of Aberdeen, Scotland.*

This is one of the ftrongeft, and moft famous chalybeate waters in Scotland. It is of the nature of our *Iflington* water, but more powerful.

PET-

PETTIGOE, *in the county of Don-*
negal, Ireland.

It is one of the ftrongeft fulphureous
waters in Ireland ; and is impregnated with vitriolated magnefia, of
which it contains near 50 grains in
the gallon.

In its virtues it refembles the *Afke-*
ron water.

PISA, *in Italy.*

About 16 miles from Pifa is a
warm bath called *Bagno a Acqua,* and
at the bottom of Mount Pifa, now
called St. Julian, 12 miles from the
town, are a number of fprings of
warm water, ufed both for drinking
and bathing.

The hotteft raifes Fahrenheit's thermometer to 104° ; the cooleft to 92°.

In fmell and tafte they differ not
from

from common water. They contain natron, fea falt, and felenite.

Thefe waters are diaphoretic and diuretic, and, if drunk in large quantity, often operate by ftool.

PLOMBIERES, *in Lorraine, France.*

The water is tepid and faponaceous, with a faltifh tafte.

It is recommended for complaints of the ftomach proceeding from acidity; in fpitting of blood; in hæmorrhages; phthifical and afthmatic complaints; in dropfy of the belly; the diabetes; fluor albus; dyfentery; and in all cutaneous diforders.

It is drunk from a pint to three quarts, on an empty ftomach, in the morning; it is diuretic and laxative.

It is alfo ufed outwardly as a bath; and is reckoned excellent for wafhing ulcers.

PONT-

PONTGIBAUT, *in Auvergne,*
France.

The water is limpid, fubacid, and
contains about 55 grains of natron,
and 50 of calcareous earth, in the
gallon.

It is diuretic and gently opening ;
and its virtues are allied to thofe of
the *Tilbury* and *Seltzer* waters.

PYRMONT, *in Weftphalia, Germany.*

This is a very brifk chalybeate, abounding in fixed air; and
when taken up from the fountain,
fparkles like the brifkeft Champaign wine. It has a fine, pleafant,
vinous tafte, and a fomewhat fulphureous fmell. It is perfectly clear,
and bears carriage better than the
Spa water.

A gal-

A gallon of it contains 46 grains of chalk, 15.6 of magnefia, 30 of vitriolated magnefia, 10 of fea falt, and 2.6 of aerated iron *.

Perfons who drink it at the well are affeated with a kind of giddinefs or intoxication; owing, it may be fuppofed, to the great quantity of fixed air with which the water abounds.

The common operation of this water is by urine; but it is alfo gently fudorific; and if taken in large quantity proves laxative. When, however, it is required to have this latter effect, it is ufual to mix fome falts with the firft glaffes.

It is drunk by glafsfuls in the morning, to the quantity of from one to five or fix pints, according to cir-

* Dr. Marcard, in his *Defcription of Pyrmont*, on the authority of M. Weftrumb of Hammeln, eftimates the iron at fomewhat more than eight grains to the gallon.

cumftances,

cumftances, walking about between each glafs.

It is recommended in cafes where the conftitution is relaxed; in want of appetite and digeftion; in weaknefs of the ftomach, and in heartburn; in the green ficknefs; in female obftructions, and in barrennefs; in the fcurvy, and cutaneous difeafes; in the gout, efpecially when mixed with milk; in cholics; in bloody fluxes; in difeafes of the breaft and lungs, in which cafes it is beft taken lukewarm; in nervous, hyfteric, and hypochondriacal diforders; in apoplexies and palfies; in the gravel, and urinary obftructions; in foulnefs of the blood; and in obftructions of the finer veffels. It amends the lax texture of the blood; exhilarates the fpirits without inflaming, as vinous liquors are apt to do; and is among the beft reftoratives in decayed and broken conftitutions.

This

This water poffeffes the general virtues of the *Spa* water; and at the fountain it is even more fpirity, as well
as a ftronger chalybeate. The reader
therefore is referred to what is faid of
the *Spa* water, for a further account of
its virtues.

To thofe to whom œconomy is an
objeét it may be of importance to
know, that the expence of living at
Pyrmont is not above half what would
be incurred at Spa.

QUEEN CAMEL, *near Wincaunton,
in Somerfetfhire.*

The water has a fœtid, fulphureous
fmell, like the wafhings of a foul gun.
It tinges filver of a yellow or black
colour, and blackens the ftones on
which it runs. It is alfo faid to be
colder than common water.

It contains natron, together with

L 6   fea

fea falt, a chalky earth, and a bituminous or fulphureous matter.

It has been ufed with fuccefs both
inwardly and outwardly in cutaneous
diforders, the fcurvy, and the King's
evil; and for thefe purpofes a place
is contrived for bathing.

RICHMOND, *in the county of Surry.*

This is a purging water, of the nature of thofe of *Acton* and *Pancras.*

RIPPON, *in Yorkſhire.*

Near this place a fpring of a pretty
ftrong fulphureous water rifes from a
limeftone hill.   A gallon yielded, on
evaporation, 66 grains, of which nearly half was earth, the remainder fea
falt.

ROAD, *in Wiltſhire.*

This is a chalybeate water with a
fulphureous fmell, and is impregnated
with natron.

It

It is recommended internally and externally in ſcorbutic and ſcrophulous caſes, and in cutaneous diſeaſes, &c.

On firſt taking this water it acts as a gentle purge.

It does not bear carriage.

ROUGHAM, *in Lancaſhire.*

It is of the nature of *Barrowdale* water, but much weaker.

The gallon contains five drams of ſea ſalt, and one dram of vitriolated magneſia.

The doſe for a purge is from three to eight quarts. In that quantity it operates powerfully by ſtool, and alſo by urine.

SAINT AMAND, *a town in French Flanders.*

There are two fountains here, one called *Bouillon* or *Bouillant*, the other

the

the fountain of *Arras*, or *L'Eveque*
d'Arras, the latter of which is the
ftrongeft.

They fomewhat refemble thofe of
Aix-la-Chapelle in appearance, but are
inferior in heat, raifing Fahrenheit's
thermometer to 75° only, when in the
open air it ftood at 50°.

They principally deferve notice on
account of the *boue* or mud baths.
The method of ufing them is to bury
the affected limb, or part of the body,
even up to the armpits, for fome hours,
as the cafe may require : the patient is
then carried to a hot bath and cleanf-
ed from the black mud which adheres
to the fkin. The *boue* is of fo firm
a confiftence that a part muft firft be
digged out. A thermometer immerfed a
foot deep in it was raifed to near 60°,
when in the open air it was at 47°. It
contains lime, magnefia and iron, all
aerared,

aerated, befides felenite, argillaceous and filiceous earth. The refiduum of the water exhibits the fame ingredients.

They both contain a peculiar air, in fmell very much refembling hepatic, which Dr. Afh attributes to a bituminous fubftance.

SAINT BARTHOLOMEW'S WELL, *Ireland. It is about two miles fouthweft from Cork.*

The water is foft, and mixes fmoothly with foap.

By keeping it putrifies, and then tinges filver, and throws up a ftinking fcum which has fomewhat of an irony tafte. Galls then give it a purple tinge, which they dō not to the frefh water.

The gallon affords 24 grains of refiduum, which is chiefly natron.

Its

Its virtues are fimilar to thofe of the *Tilbury* water.

SAINT ERASMUS'S WELL, *fi-tuated on Lord Chetwynd's grounds in Staffordfhire.*

The water is of the nature of *Bar-rowdale*, but much weaker, the gallon yielding only four drams 32 grains of fea falt.

It is of the colour of fack, but without much tafte or fmell.

If drunk to the quantity of feveral quarts, it operates powerfully by ftool.

SALES SPA.

See *Lancafter.*

SCARBOROUGH, *in Yorkfhire.*

The waters of this place are chalybeate and purging; and they are more frequented and ufed than any other water of this clafs in England.

There

There are two wells; the one more purgative, the other a ftronger cha-lybeate. Hence the latter (which is neareft the town) has been called the *chalybeate* fpring, the other the *purging*; though they are both impregnated with the fame principles, but in dif-ferent proportions. The *purging* is the moft famed, and is that which is ufually called the *Scarborough* water. This contains 52 grains of calcareous earth, two of ochre, and 266 of vi-triolated magnefia, in the gallon: the chalybeate, 70 grains of calcareous earth, 139 of vitriolated magnefia, and 11 of fea falt.

When thefe waters are poured out of one glafs into another, they throw up a number of air-bubbles; and if fhaken for a while in a clofe ftopt phial, and the phial be fuddenly opened be-fore the commotion ceafes, they dif-plode

plode an elaſtic vapour with an audible noiſe, which ſhows that they abound in fixed air.

At the fountain they both have a briſk, pungent, chalybeate taſte; but the *purging* water taſtes bitteriſh, which is not uſually the caſe with the *chalybeate* one.

They loſe their chalybeate virtues by expoſure, and alſo by keeping; but the purging water ſooneſt.

They both putrify by keeping; but in time recover their ſweetneſs.

Four or five half pints of the *purging* water drunk within an hour, give two or three eaſy motions, and raiſe the ſpirits. The like quantity of the *chalybeate* purges leſs, but exhilarates more, and paſſes off chiefly by urine.

Theſe waters have been found of ſervice in hectic fevers, in weakneſſes of the ſtomach, and indigeſtion; in

relaxations

relaxations of the fyftem; in nervous, hyfteric, and hypochondriacal diforders; in the green ficknefs, in the fcurvy, rheumatifm, and afthmatic complaints; in gleets, the fluor albus, and other preternatural evacuations, and in habitual coftivenefs. The waters are to be varied according to the intention to be anfwered.

S C O L L I E N S E S, *in Upper Rhoetia,* *Switzerland.*

It is a chalybeate water, impregnated with natron; and fo full of fixed air, that it often burfts the bottles in which it is kept.

It makes the drinkers giddy, and operates mildly, though largely, by ftool, and by fpitting.

It is efteemed excellent for cholic y pains, both as a cure and preventative.

In

In its general virtues it refembles the *Spa* water.

Sea Water.

Sea water has a falt, bitterifh tafte, appears of a greenifh colour, and be-comes fœtid by keeping.

As an immenfe number of fprings, rivers, &c. are continually emptying themfelves into the fea, as it contains an almoft infinity of animals and ve-getables, and covers and wafhes fuch a variety of lands and fhores, it would feem to be impregnated with very hete-rogeneous matters. Neverthelefs, the water, in different parts of the ocean, appears to be nearly alike, and the difference in its contents to be much lefs than might at firft be imagined.

A gallon, taken up off Brighthelm-ftone, 400 yards from low-water mark,

yielded

yielded three ounces 323$\frac{1}{2}$ grains of
fea falt, one ounce 283$\frac{3}{4}$ grains of muriated magnefia, and 93$\frac{1}{4}$ grains of
gypfum. It alfo afforded one ounce
meafure of fixed air, four of atmofpheric, and one of phlogifticated.

Sea water, in hotter climates, generally contains a greater proportion of
thefe matters than that in colder ones,
and therefore is ftronger. The difference, in fome places, is above two
to one.

Sea water taken internally, in a fmall
quantity, proves a ftimulating and
heating remedy, diffipating the finer
fluids, and occafioning thirft.

In a larger quantity it proves purgative. But differs from other purges
in that patients who drink it daily for
a confiderable time, inftead of lofing,
often gain ftrength by it.

It therefore acts not merely as a
purgative, but gives alfo a brifk ftimulus

mulus to the ftomach and inteftines, thereby increafing the appetite, and promoting digeftion.

By means of this excellent property of fea water (viz. our being able to keep up a purging for a confiderable time, without hurting the conftitution) we are enabled frequently to remove diforders which have refifted the force of other remedies.

It is of excellent ufe in fcrophulous complaints; and glandular fwellings are generally removed by it. If joined with the bark, it has fometimes a better effect in thofe cafes.

It is alfo ferviceable in purging off grofs humours, which have been the confequence of indulging the appetite too freely, and leading an inactive life : alfo in cleanfing the inteftines of vifcid mucus, and worms.

In cafes where there is fever, heat, or inflammation, fea water is found to

be

✝

be hurtful. Previous to its ufe, there-fore, thefe fymptoms fhould be re-moved by bleeding, purging, and a proper cooling treatment.

As fea water is fpecifically heavier than common water, and (by reafon of the faline matters contained in it) is alfo more ftimulating, it is more efficacious when ufed externally as a bath.

It has alfo particular virtues when externally ufed.. On account of its ftimulating and difcutient property, it is excellent in the fcrophula or king's evil, in hard fwellings, in the bite of a mad dog, in the rickets, in the dry leprofy and itch, in paralytic and fcorbutic complaints, and in many other cafes. But in moft of thefe, it is proper to ufe it both internally and externally.

S E D

SEDLITZ, *Germany,* *a village in*
Bohemia.

This purging water is of the fame
nature as our Epfom, but much
ftronger, a gallon yielding about two
ounces of the purging falt.

Two or three tea-cups full are generally fufficient for a dofe; and the
ftrongeft conftitution fcarce requires
more than a pint.

SELTZER, *in Germany.* *This Spring*
is near to the town of Neider, or
Lower Seltzer, about three leagues
from Franckfort on the Maine, in
the Lower Archbifhoprick of Treves.

It rifes near a fmall trout ftream.
The country and avenues around are
delightful, and afford a very pleafing
profpect.

The water iffues forth with great
rapidity;

rapidity; is remarkably clear and light, and on pouring it from one veſſel to another, plenty of air-bubbles ariſe.

It has, at firſt, ſomewhat of a briſk ſubacid pungent taſte, but leaves behind a lixivial one.

If expoſed twenty-four hours to the air, it loſes entirely its original taſte, and acquires that of a flat alkaline ley. But no ſediment is depoſited.

It putrifies ſooner than any other medicinal water.

When freſh, it makes an immediate effervefcence with acids, but eſpecially with Rheniſh wines, and a little powdered ſugar.

It alſo curdles with a ſolution of ſoap.

It does not change purple with galls; and therefore contains no chalybeate.

Oil of tartar dropt into it makes it milky, but does not occaſion a precipitate.

M   It

It contains 14 grains of chalk, 20½ of magnefia, 141.6 of natron, and 92 of fea falt, in the gallon. From this quantity of the water 128 ounce meafures of fixed air were obtained.

Its operation is chiefly by urine, for it has no purgative virtues. It corrects acidities, renders the blood and juices more fluid, and promotes a brifk and free circulation. Hence it is good in obftructions of the glands, and againft grofs and vifcid humours.

It is of great ufe in the gravel and ftone, and in other diforders of the kidnies and bladder.

It is alfo excellent in gouty and rheumatic complaints*, efpecially when mixed with milk †.

* In thefe diforders its virtue is faid to be much improved by the addition of Rhenifh wine, and a little fugar.

† Affes, or goats milk, is ufually preferred.

It

It is drunk with great fuccefs in fcorbutic, cutaneous, and putrid diforders.

It is good againft the heart-burn; and it is alfo an excellent ftomachic. Several pints may be drunk in the courfe of a day.

On account of its diuretic quality, it is of fervice in dropfical complaints.

Mixed with affes milk, it is of great ufe in confumptive cafes, and in diforders of the lungs.

It is in great efteem in nervous diforders, either with, or without milk, as is found to be moft fuitable to the conftitution.

It is alfo of fervice in hypochondriacal and hyfteric complaints, and in obftructions of the menfes, efpecially if exercife be ufed.

It is given in purgings and fluxes arifing from acidity in the bowels, with good fuccefs.

M 2 Drunk

Drunk by nurſes, it is ſaid to render their milk more wholeſome and
nouriſhing to children, and to prevent it from turning ſour on their
ſtomachs.

As the fixed air of this water ſo
ſoon flies off, it ought either to be
drunk on the ſpot, or at leaſt ſhould
be impregnated with a freſh quantity
previous to its being taken, according
to the directions given in the beginning of this treatiſe.

Thoſe perſons, with whoſe ſtomachs water alone does not ſo well
agree, are adviſed to mix with it ſome
generous and agreeable wine, in caſes
where wine will not be hurtful. (See
alſo *Spa* and *Pyrmont* waters).

S E N E, or S E N D, *near the Devizes,*
Wiltſhire.

At this place are two chalybeate
ſprings, one of them ſtronger than
the

the other, but both refembling in virtues the *Hampftead* and *Iflington* waters.

They are diuretic, but not purgative.

At a village called *Paulfholt,* near
this place, is another chalybeate
fpring.

S E Y D S C H U T Z, *in Germany.*

It is fituated near to that of *Sedlitz,*
and is of the fame purgative nature,
but fomewhat ftronger.

S H A D W E L L, *near London, fituated in Sun Tavern Fields.*

This is a vitriolic chalybeate water, and is one of the ftrongeft waters
of the kind in England; it alfo contains iron held in folution by aerial
acid. The gallon yielded 1132 grains

M 3   of

of martial vitriol, and 188 of an ochry-coloured earth.

It has an acid, auftere, vitriolic tafte, and with galls gives a blueifh black colour like ink.

It has been taken inwardly to the quantity of a pint, divided into two or three dofes in the courfe of an hour in the morning. It vomits, and gently purges; it turns the ftools black.

It has been found of fervice in the fluor albus, in obftinate gleets, and dyfenteries; in inward bleedings; in the jaundice; and in fcorbutic and leprous cafes. But it has chiefly been ufed externally for fore eyes, the itch, fcabs, tetters, fcald-head, ulcers, fiftulas, and the like, by wafhing, or elfe applying linen rags dipped in it to the parts.

In fcorbutic and leprous cafes, the internal ufe is firft advifed till the

eruptions

eruptions are thrown out, which are then to be removed by the outward application of the water.

SHAPMOOR. *The Spring is situated in a marshy heath, between Shap and Orton, in Westmoreland.*

This is a sulphureous water, impregnated with a purging salt, composed of vitriolated magnesia, sea salt, and natron, about 370 grains in the gallon.

Three pints of it prove purgative.

In its virtues it seems to resemble the *Askeron* water.

SHETTLEWOOD, *situated between Bolsover and Romeley, in Derbyshire.*

It is a sulphureous water, containing near two drams of sea salt in the gallon.

M 4 Its

Its virtues refemble thofe of the *Harrogate* water.

SHIPTON, *in Yorkfhire.*

It is a fulphureous water, impregnated with fea falt, together with a purging falt.

In its virtues it refembles the *Harrogate* water.

SOMERSHAM, *in Huntingdonfhire.*

This is a chalybeate water, impregnated with green vitriol and alum, and contains alfo fixed air.

The feafon for drinking it is from May to October.

It is drunk in the morning to the quantity of feveral glaffes. It is recommended in debilities of the ftomach and bowels, in dyfenteries, hæmorrhoids, and worms, in nidorous crudities, in obftructions of the liver and fpleen,

in

in uterine complaints, in the ftone and gravel, in the fcurvy, in hyfteric and hypochondriacal diforders, and many others.

It is proper to purge before and after the courfe, and falts may alfo be occafionally added to it.

Externally it is applied to foul ulcers and cancers.

Spa, *in the bifhoprick of Liege, Germany, twenty-one miles fouth-eaft from the town of Liege.*

In and about this town there are feveral fprings, which afford excellent chalybeate waters: and in Great Britain they are the moft drunk of any foreign mineral waters.

The principal fprings are,

1. The Pohoun, or Pouhon, fituated in the middle of the village.
2. Sauviniere, about a mile and a half eaft from it.

3. Grois-

3. GROISBEECK, near to the Sauviniere.
4. TONNELET, a little to the left of
   the road to the Sauviniere.
5. WATROZ, near to the Tonnelet.
6. GERONSTERE, two miles fouth
   of the Spa.
7. SARTS, or NIVERSET, in the diftrict of Sarts.
8. CHEVRON, or BRU, in the principality of Stavelot.
9. COUVE,
10. BEVERSEE, } All near Malmdy.
11. SIGE,
12. GEROMONT.

The POUHON is a flow deep fpring,
and is more or lefs ftrong or gafeous
according to the ftate of the atmofphere.

The gallon contains 10 grains of
chalk, 30 of magnefia, 10 of natron,
and five of aerated iron. It yields of
fixed air 132 ounce meafures.

It

It contains more iron than either of the other fprings, and does not fo foon lofe its gas.

It is in its moft perfect and natural ftate in cold, dry weather. It then appears colourlefs, tranfparent, and without fmell, and has a fubacid cha-lybeate tafte, with an agreeable fmart-nefs: at fuch times, if it be taken out of the well in a glafs, it does not fparkle; but after ftanding awhile, covers the glafs on the infide with fmall air-bubbles; but if it be fhaken, or poured out of one glafs into an-other, it then fparkles, and difcharges a great number of air-bubbles at the furface.

In warm, moift weather, it lofes its tranfparency, appears turbid or wheyifh, contains lefs fixed air, and is partly decompofed. A murmuring

noife

noife alfo is fometimes heard in the well.

It is colder than the heat of the atmofphere by many degrees.

It is fuppofed to contain the greateft quantity of fixed air of almoft any acidulous water; and in confequence thereof has a remarkable fprightlinefs and vinofity, and boils by mere warmth. This, however, foon flies off, if the water be left expofed; though in well corked bottles it is in a great meafure preferved.

It is capable of diffolving more iron than it naturally contains, and thereby becoming a ftronger chalybeate. This is owing to the great quantity of fixed air which it contains.

For the fame reafon an ebullition is raifed in this water on the addition of acids, as they difengage its fixed air.

It

It mixes fmoothly with milk, whether it be cold or of a boiling heat.

Of the Sauvinière water, a gallon yields 6.5 grains of chalk, 4.5 of magnefia, two of natron, 3.5 of kali, 2.2 of aerated iron, and 108 ounce meafures of fixed air.

At the well it has fomewhat a fmell of fulphur.

Groisbeeck. The water is of the fame nature as the Sauviniere, but contains a fomewhat larger proportion of the feveral ingredients. It has a vitriolic tafte, and fomewhat of a fulphureous fmell.

Tonnelet. This is one of the moft fprightly waters in the world. It is much colder than either of the other Spa waters; has no fmell; is bright, tranfparent, and colourlefs; and from the rapidity of its motion does not foul its bafon. It has a fmart, fubacid,

fprightly

fprightly tafte, not unlike the brifkeft
Champaign wine.

From a variety of experiments it
appears, that this water is more ftrongly charged than any of the others with
fixed air, on which the *energy* of all
waters of this kind depends, but it parts
with it more readily.

It contains more iron than either
of the fprings, except the Pouhon.

WATROZ. Its fituation is loweft
of any of the fprings about Spa, and
it is more apt to be foul: but when the
well is cleaned out, and the water
pure, it is found to be of the fame
nature as that of POUHON. It is not
purgative, as fome have afferted.

GERONSTERE. This water has
much lefs fixed air than the POUHON.
It has a fulphureous fmell at the fountain, which it lofes by being carried
to a diftance. This fmell is ftrongeft
in warm moift weather.

The

The air, or vapour, of this water affects the heads of some who drink it, occafioning a giddinefs, or kind of drunkennefs, which goes off in a quarter or half an hour. The Pyrmont, and feveral other brifk chalybeate waters, are found to have the fame effect.

It is colder than any of the fprings, the *Tonnelet* excepted.

SARTS, or NIVERSET. It refembles the *Tonnelet* water, but is rather lefs brifk and gafeous. It is however more acid and ftyptic.

BRU, or CHEVRON. The phyficians at Liege have artfully decried this water, becaufe it is not in the principality of Liege. But by every trial it appears not much inferior to any of the *Spa* waters. In the quantity of fixed air and of iron it contains, it approaches the Pouhon.

COUVE and BEVERSEE. The *Couve* nearly refembles the *Tonnelet* water;

4 or

or rather, may be placed in a medium between that and the *Watroz*. It hardly equals the tranfparency, fmartnefs, and generous vinous tafte of the firft, but it greatly furpaffes the latter. The *Beverfee* agrees with this, only that it does not retain its fmartnefs fo well by keeping.

LA SIGE. It has fome of the general properties of the *Spa* waters, but in other refpects it is different.

It is moderately fubacid, fmart, and grateful, but has no fenfible chalybeate tafte.

It fparkles like Champaign wine when poured from one glafs to another. Upon ftanding it lofes its fixed air, and throws up a thick mother-of-pearl coloured pellicle.

It is much more loaded with earthy matters, and lefs impregnated with iron and fixed air, than the other Spa waters.

GEROMONT. As a chalybeate and acidu-

acidulous water it feems to be nearly of the fame ftrength with *La Sige*; but it contains a greater quantity of natron, together with a mixture of fea falt. The earthy matters, however, are lefs.

Their Virtues, &c.—It appears, that thefe waters are compounded of nearly the fame principles, though in different proportions. All of them abound with *fixed air*. They contain more or lefs iron, natron, and calcareous and felenitical earths; together with a fmall portion of fea falt, and an oily matter common to all waters. Thefe are all kept fufpended, and in a neutral ftate, by means of the aerial acid, or fixed air.

From a review of the contents of thefe waters, it cannot be imagined that their virtues principally depend on the fmall quantity of *folid* matters which they contain. They muft

there-

therefore depend moſtly on their ſub-
tle mineral ſpirit, or *fixed air*. And
they are probably rendered more ac-
tive and penetrating both in the firſt
paſſages, and alſo when they enter the
circulation, by means of that ſmall
portion of iron, earth, ſalt, &c. with
which they are impregnated.

Theſe waters are diuretic, and ſometimes purgative; like other chalybeate
waters they tinge the ſtools black.

They exhilarate and affect the ſpirits with a much more kind and be-
nign influence than wine or ſpirituous
liquors; and their general operation
is by ſtrengthening the fibres.   They
cool and quench thirſt much better
than common water.

They are therefore found excellent
in caſes of univerſal languor or weakneſs, proceeding from a relaxation of
the ſtomach; and of the fibres in general, and where the conſtitution has
been

been weakened by difeafe, or by too
fedentary a life. In weak, relaxed,
grofs habits; in nervous diforders; in
the end of the gout and rheumatifm,
where the conftitution needs to be re-
paired; in fuch afthmatic diforders and
chronic coughs as proceed from too
great a relaxation of the pulmonary
veffels; in obftruçtions of the liver
and fpleen; in cafes where the blood
is too thin and putrefcent, occafioned
by irregularities, or by fcorbutic or
other putrid diforders; in hyfterical
and hypochondriacal complaints, where
the fibres are too irritable and relaxed, and where the habit in general
needs to be reftored; in paralytic diforders; in gleets; in the fluor albus;
in fluxes of the belly; and in other
inordinate difcharges proceednig from
too great weaknefs or relaxation of
any particular part; in the gravel and
ftone; in female obftruçtions; in barrennefs;

rennefs; and in moft other cafes where a ftrengthening and brifk ftimulating refolving chalybeate remedy is wanted; and where there are no confirmed obftructions, or fo much heat and fever as to forbid their ufe.

They are, however, generally hurtful in hot, bilious, and plethoric conftitutions, when ufed before the body is cooled by proper evacuations. They are alfo hurtful in cafes of fever and heat; in hectic fevers and ulcerations of the lungs, and of other internal parts, particularly where there is no free outlet to the matter; and alfo in moft confirmed obftructions attended with fever.

The ufual feafon for drinking them is in July and Auguft, or during the fummer months from May to September. The water, however, is beft in the winter, and in dry, frofty weather;

ther; and probably might then be drunk to greateſt advantage.

If they lie cold on the ſtomach, a few carraway ſeeds, cardamoms, or other aromatic, may be taken with them. The veſſel out of which it is drunk may alſo be warmed with hot water, or a little warm water may be added immediately before drinking. It muſt always be drunk before noon.

The quantity to be drunk ſhould be different according to the age, conſtitution, and other circumſtances of the patient. The only certain rule is, that quantity which the ſtomach can bear without heavineſs or uneaſineſs. The greater the quantity any one drinks, the. better, provided it agrees, and paſſes well off. It is adviſeable to begin with drinking a glaſs or two ſeveral times in a day, increaſing the quantity daily, as far as the ſtomach will bear. To continue that doſe du-

ring

ring the courfe, and to finifh by lef-
fening it by the fame degrees by which
it was augmented.   Moderate exercife is proper after drinking.   It is to
be continued for feveral weeks or
months, according to the circumftances.

Previous to the ufe of the water, it
is proper to cleanfe the firft paffages
by gentle purges, and if judged neceffary, an emetic alfo fhould be given.   During the courfe, likewife,
coftivenefs fhould be prevented, by occafionally adding Rochelle falts, or
rhubarb, to the firft glaffes of water
in the morning.

When there is too much heat, the
faline draughts, nitre, vegetable acids,
or the like, fhould be given; and the
elixir of vitriol has been added to the
water, in intermittent feverifh complaints, with good effect.

A cooling regimen fhould be obferved

ed while drinking thefe waters, as alfo
regular hours, and quietnefs, or chear-
fulnefs of mind.

In cafes of rigidity of the fibres,
the warm bath is recommended,
among the beft preparatives to a courfe
of thefe waters; and, hence bathing
at *Aix-la-Chapelle,* or at *Chaude Fon-
taine,* is often premifed. The warm
bathing may occafionally be repeated
during the courfe. In oppofite cafes,
the cold bath is recommended.

The Spa water is ufed alfo externally, in a variety of cafes, with good
fuccefs. It is ufed as an injection in
the fluor albus, and in ulcers and cancers of the womb, and alfo in the go-
norrhœa; it is ferviceable in venereal
aphthæ, and ulcers in the mouth; it
is ufed to wafh phagedenic ulcers; it is
recommended by way of gargle for relaxed tonfils, and for faftening loofe
teeth; it is alfo good in other relaxations;

tions; and it is faid to cure the itch, and fimilar complaints, by wafhing and bathing, an internal courfe being alfo obferved at the time.

As the Spa waters are impregnated with different proportions of the fame ingredients, they may be chofen differently, according to the intentions we have in view. The *Pohoun* is the ftrongeft chalybeate. The *Tonnelet* is a weaker chalybeate, but brifker, and rather more gafeous. The *Groif-beeck* and *Sauviniere* are ftill weaker chalybeates, but contain a portion of kali, which the others do not. The *Geromont* is likewife a weak chalybeate, but contains a great deal of calcareous and felenitical earth, and about three times as much alkaline falt as any of the others. The four laft waters, therefore, will be better in diforders arifing from an acid caufe, and as diuretics, particularly the *Geromont*.

STANGER, *near Cockermouth, in Cumberland.*

This is a falt chalybeate, or vitriolic water; and, when drunk to four or five pints, operates with violence both upwards and downwards.

STENFIELD, *in Lincolnſhire.*

It is a chalybeate laxative water, and refembles that of *Orſton.* It is light, clear, pleafant tafted, and full of gas at firſt, but on long ſtanding in its large refervoir fpoils.

STREATHAM, *in Surry, near London.*

The water has a yellowiſh tinge, and throws up a fcum variegated with blue, green, and yellow. Its taſte is fomewhat faline and difagreeable.

N The

The gallon contains 160 grains of falt compofed of fea falt and vitriolated magnefia, and 40 of calcareous earth.

It is a mild purging water, and may be drunk to the quantity of three or four pints.

It is alfo diuretic, and is faid to be found ufeful in diforders of the eyes.

S T O K E.

See *Jeſſop's Well.*

S U C H A L O Z A, *about a mile from Hungarian Broda, in Germany.*

It is an acidulous water, refembling that of *Nezdenice* in virtues.

It is greatly efteemed in the neighbourhood for the cure of fcrophulous and other diforders, in which waters of this kind are ferviceable; and is

drunk

drunk with victuals inftead of fmall beer and wine.

SUTTON BOG, *in the county of Ox-ford, near to Northamptonſhire.*

This is one of the waters termed *ſulphureous.*

It has an intolerable fœtid fmell, like rotten eggs. Its tafte is faltiſh and pungent, like foap lees.

It throws up a blue fcum, and the mud at the bottom is jet black. In half an hour it turns filver of a cop-per colour.

It contains 131 grains of natron mixed with a little fea falt, and nine grains of argillaceous earth, in the gal-lon.

It is a mild laxative, or purging water.

It is ufed both for drinking and bathing; and ulcers, tumours, fcro-

phulous,

phulous, and other difeafes of the
fkin, are fuccefsfully wafhed with it.
The mud is alfo made ufe of.

SWADLINGBAR, *in the county of*
Cavan, Ireland.

The water is fometimes tranfparent and colourlefs; at other times
fomewhat whitifh.

It has a ftrong fulphureous fmell,
which it retains long in bottles well
corked.   It tinges filver of a blackifh
or copperifh colour.

The well is commonly covered
with a whitifh or blueifh fcum; and
depofits a mud which burns, on a red
hot iron, with a blue flame.

It contains natron, together with a
little vitriolated magnefia and earth.

SWANSEY, *in Glamorganfhire,*
North Wales.

It is impregnated with vitriolated
iron,

iron, of which a gallon yields thirty-two grains.

Dr. Rutty fufpects it to contain copper.

Taken inwardly it is alfo faid to ftop purgings; applied outwardly it ftops bleeding.

SYDENHAM, *in Kent, near London.*

The water is fomewhat bitterifh to the tafte.

It is purgative, and of the nature of *Epfom* water, but only about half the ftrength of it.

TARLETON, *eight miles from Pref-ton, in Lancafhire.*

This is a chalybeate water, and drunk to the quantity of three or four pints proves purgative. In its virtues it feems to refemble the *Scarborough* water.

N 3 It

It has a fomewhat fulphureous fmell when firft drawn.

TEWKESBURY, *in Gloucefterfhire.*

It is a purging water, of the nature of thofe of *Acton, Pancras,* and *Epfom.*

There are two other fprings of the fame kind in the neighbourhood; one of them is in Walton grounds*, the other in Teddington grounds.

THETFORD, *in the county of Norfolk.*

This is a chalybeate and acidulous water, and contains alfo natron.

It operates by urine, and alfo gently by ftool.

It is recommended in pains of the ftomach and bowels; in lofs of appetite; in relaxed ftate of the fibres; in

* See *Walton.*

hyfteric

hyſteric diſorders; and in beginning conſumptions.

THOROTON, *near Newark upon Trent, Nottinghamſhire.*

It is a chalybeate laxative water, reſembling that of *Orſton.*

THURSK, *in the North Riding of Yorkſhire.*

It is a briſk, ſparkling, chalybeate water, and is alſo purgative and diu-retic. It reſembles the *Scarborough* and *Cheltenham* waters.

TIBSHELF, *in Derbyſhire.*

This is a fine clear chalybeate; and when poured from one glaſs to an-other, ſparkles like the *Spa* water, which it reſembles in virtues.

TIL-

TILBURY. *The Spring which affords this water is fituated near a farm-houfe at Weft-Tilbury, near Tilbury-Fort, in Effex.*

This water is not quite limpid at the well, but is fomewhat ftraw-coloured.

It is foft and fmooth to the tafte; though after being agitated in the mouth, it leaves a fmall degree of roughnefs on the tongue.

It throws up a fcum variegated with feveral colours, which feels greafy, and effervefces with vitriolic acid.

It mixes fmooth with milk, but curdles with foap. When boiled it turns milky; a fourth part of mountain wine fines it immediately, and all acids do the fame.

A gallon of the water contains 37 grains

grains of chalk, 49 of true nitre, 82 of fea falt, and $1\frac{1}{2}$ of natron.

It operates chiefly by urine, though it is alfo fomewhat purgative; and increafes perfpiration.

It is in efteem for removing glandular obftructions; it is good in bloody fluxes, purgings, and the like; in diforders of the ftomach arifing from acidity; in the gravel; fluor albus; and immoderate flux of the menfes.

As a diuretic it is good in dropfical complaints.

It gently warms the ftomach, ftrengthens the appetite, and promotes digeftion; it is alfo of fervice in lownefs of fpirits. From its efficacy in removing obftructions of the glands, it is recommended in fcurvies and cutaneous difeafes; and its virtues in thefe complaints feem to be confirmed by the tingling which it occafions in the fkin.

The dofe is ufually a quart in a day.

TOBER

TOBER BONY, *in Ireland.*

This fpring is fituated about four miles north of Dublin.

The water is fweet, and foon lathers with foap.

Before rain and wind it yields a fœtid fmell. Its fediment, when placed on hot iron, turns black and fœtid.

It contains an alkaline falt, together with a calcareous earth, and an oily or bituminous matter.

Its virtues are fimilar to thofe of the *Tilbury* water, but in a lefs degree.

TONSTEIN, *in the Bifhoprick of Cologne, Germany.*

This is among the moft noted waters of Germany.

The water has a brifk fubacid tafte at the fountain, which is loft by expofure to the air.

It

It is clear and limpid when taken up from the well, but becomes turbid by ftanding; owing to the lofs of its fixed air.

It contains a chalky earth with an alkali and a little fea falt.

Its virtues are fimilar to thofe of the *Seltzer* waters, but it is more purgative.

It may alfo be ufed with advantage for common drink, either by itfelf or mixed with wine; and that either in acute or chronic difeafes, where diuretic or deobftruent remedies are required.

T o w n l e y.

See *Hanbridge.*

T r a l e e, *in the county of Kerry, Ireland.*

It is a chalybeate water, of the nature of that of *Caftleconnel.*

Tun-

TUNBRIDGE. *The* WELLS *are fi-*
tuated about five miles from the town
of Tunbridge, in Kent.

This is at prefent one of the moft
famous chalybeate waters in England,
and the moft reforted to of any, tho'
it does not feem to be preferable to
many others in this kingdom.

It is a brifk, light water, has a ferruginous tafte, and contains alfo a little
fea falt.

Expofed to the air it foon lofes its
virtues; as it does alfo in a few days
in bottles.

It is ufual at times to mix with the
firft glafs of the water, taken in the
morning, either a little common falt,
or fome other purging falt, in order to
make it operate by ftool. If the ftomach be foul, it is apt to vomit.

It is chiefly reforted to in June,
July,

July, and Auguſt; and is recommended in all thoſe diſorders in which
the celebrated *Spa waters of Germany*
are ſerviceable. It poſſeſſes the ſame
general virtues as thoſe waters, but in
a leſs degree.

UPMINSTER, *near Brentwood, in Eſſex.*

This is a ſtrong ſulphureous water, impregnated with a purging ſalt,
and natron.

It retains its ſulphureous quality a
long time.

It is purgative and diuretic; and
in its virtues ſeems to reſemble the
Aſkeron water.

VAHLS, *in France.*

The well is near Vahls, in Dau-
phiny.

The water has a briſk ſubacid taſte
at the ſpring; which is loſt before it
reaches

reaches Paris, for it then taftes faltifh.

It contains 455 grains of natron in
the gallon.

It is diuretic, and fomewhat purgative; and is fimilar in virtues to
the *Seltzer* and *Clifton* waters, though
lefs powerful.

N. B. Near to this is another fpring,
called *La Marie*, of the fame kind, but
weaker.

W A L T O N, *near Tewkefbury.*

This water contains the fame ingredients as that of *Cheltenham*. The
only difference between them confifts
in the quantity of the purging falt
in the latter being fomewhat greater,
whilft the *Walton* water has rather
more hepatic air.

W A R D R E W, *in Northumberland.*

It is fituated between Cumberland
and

and Northumberland, on the banks of the river Arden.

It is the moſt cold ſulphureous water in the three northren counties. It contains ſea ſalt, and therefore reſembles in virtues the *Harrogate* water. The ſalt is in the proportion of about 22 grains to the gallon.

It loſes both its ſmell and virtues by carriage and keeping.

WEATHERSTACK, *in Weſtmoreland.*

This is a weak chalybeate water, but contains a large portion of ſea ſalt. In the ſummer it ſmells of ſulphur, but not in the winter.

It is purgative; and the doſe is two or three pints.

WELLENBROW, *in Northamptonſhire.*

It is a ſlight· chalybeate water, reſembling that of *Iſlington.*

WEST

§

WEST ASHTON, *in the parifh of Steeple Afhton, Wiltfhire.*

It is a weak chalybeate water, re-fembling thofe of *Iflington* and *Tun-bridge.*

WESTWOOD, *near Tanderfley, in Derbyfhire.*

This is a vitriolic chalybeate, fome-what refembling the *Shadwell* water.

It is recommended externally for old fores in the legs.

N. B. The coal waters, in general, in this part of the country, are alfo vitriolic.

WEXFORD, *in Ireland.*

It is an agreeable chalybeate wa-ter, fimilar in virtue to that of *Ifling-ton.*

WHITE-

WHITE-ACRE, *near Trales, in Lancashire.*

This is a very clear, brisk chalybeate water, resembling that of *Lancaster* in virtues, but it is said rather to bind than purge.

WIGAN, *in Lancashire.*

It is a clear chalybeate water, resembling those of *Hampstead* and *Islington.*

From the bottom rises an inflammable vapour, which takes fire at the surface on the approach of a lighted candle.

WIGGLESWORTH, *in the parish of Long Preston, in the West Riding of Yorkshire, four miles south of Settle.*

The water is very black, and has a
strong

ftrong fulphureous fmell, with a faltifh tafte.

Drunk to the quantity of three
quarts it purges, and two quarts are
faid to vomit, though it is rather un-
common that more fhould be required for the former than for the latter.

WILDUNGAN, *in the country of* *Waldeck, Germany.*

This water at the fountain has a
brifk fubacid tafte, which it lofes by
expofure.

It is of the fame kind with that of
Buch, but weaker.

It is one of the mildeft acidulæ
known, and may be ufed as common
drink alone, or mixed with a fmall
portion of wine.

Though it is not efteemed ftrong
enough to remove obftinate chronic
difeafes, and clear the firft paffages,
yet

yet it is excellent for blunting and di-
luting acrid, fcorbutic, and gouty humours, when taken in large quantity,
and for a fufficient length of time.

WIRKSWORTH, *in Derbyſhire.*

It is a weak fulphureous water,
impregnated with a purging falt, and
is alfo chalybeate.

It is recommended in fcrophulous,
and cutaneous diforders.

WITHAM, *in Eſſex.*

This is a chalybeate water of confiderable ftrength, and is alfo impregnated with fea falt, but it will not
bear carriage, and muft be drunk at
the fountain.

It is very diuretic, and has been
fuccefsfully prefcribed in hectic fevers, in weaknefs occafioned by long
difeafe, in lownefs of fpirits, nervous
com-

complaints, want of appetite, indigeſtion, habitual cholic, and vomiting;
in agues, in the jaundice, and beginning dropſy; in the gravel, and in
aſthmatic and ſcorbutic diſorders.

ZAHOROVICE, *in Germany.*

The ſpring is near to this village,
in the diſtrict of the Caſtle of Suiet-
lovia, in a rocky valley, by the ſide
of the river Nezdenice.

It is an acidulous water, ſalter, but
leſs acid than that of *Nezdenice*; and
it is alſo ſomewhat pungent and fœtid.

It is in great eſteem in the neighbourhood, particularly for the cure of
ſcrophulous diſorders.

CON-

CONCLUSION.

FOR the fake of brevity, I have omitted a particular defcription of each water in the preceding account, and occafionally referred the reader to fome water of the fame kind which has been more fully treated of; and the general virtues of the different claffes of waters are alfo defcribed at large in the Introduction.

In the Appendix to Dr. Prieftley's tract, I have given directions for imitating fome of thofe waters. The acidulous waters of the 5th clafs, for example, may be imitated, and even excelled, by fimply impregnating water with *Fixed Air*. The folid ingredients are known to be of little or no confequence. If, however, thefe be defired,

fired, they may be added in the proportions directed under the article *Seltzer
water*; though it is by no means neceffary that thofe proportions fhould
be ftrictly adhered to.

A purging water, anfwering perhaps all the intentions of thofe of the
6th clafs, may be made as directed for
the *Seidfcutz water*. Rochelle falt,
or vitriolated natron, may be fubftituted for the vitriolated magnefia, if
the latter be too naufeous ; and a little common falt may alfo be added.
If the water to be imitated be a falt
water, like that of the fea, the common falt fhould be in the greater proportion.

The chalybeate waters of the 1ft
clafs may be elegantly fubftituted, by
water impregnated with Fixed Air, in
which iron-filings, or wire, has been
infufed: or they may be made as directed under the articles *Spa* and *Pyrmont
water*.

water. The chalybeate purging waters of the 2d clafs may be imitated by adding to a gallon of this water two or three ounces of vitriolated magnefia, or other purging falt, and, if you will, a little fea falt.

For the fulphureous waters of the 3d clafs, water impregnated with hepatic air may be advantageoufly ufed : or they may be made as directed under the article *Aix-la-Chapelle water.* If they be alfo required to be chalybeate, or purging, or both, iron-filings, or vitriolated magnefia, or both thefe, may be added, together with a little fea falt, according to circumftances. For cold fulphureous waters, both fixed and hepatic airs are to be employed, as mentioned in the Appendix ; and even for the hot fulphureous waters it may be proper to put a fmall proportion of chalk with the fulphurated

rated kali into the lower veffel A of the apparatus.

They who have a knowledge of natural philofophy, will perceive that thefe artificial waters are not only equal, but even fuperior to the natural ones, efpecially when they cannot be drunk at the fpring head. Their virtues, for the moft part, depend on their *volatile* principles, and art can make water imbibe more than double the quantity of fixed, or hepatic air, that the ftrongeft natural waters are ever found to contain. The latter are alfo frequently impregnated with hurtful, or, at leaft, ufelefs ingredients; and we cannot always be fure that we have them genuine. It is not, however, by any means, the Author's wifh to profcribe the ufe of the natural waters. Many of them have particular virtues, as has been proved by un-

doubted

doubted experiments : and there are others which art cannot yet fufficiently imitate.

Many people again, through prejudice, will not ufe the artificial waters, as they do not believe it poffible that they can be made fufficiently to refemble the natural ones ; but even thefe will not object to the ufe of water impregnated with *fixed* or *hepatic air* in a *medicinal* view.

Water impregnated with fixed air is now known to be a very powerful antifeptic, or corrector of putrefaction. It will preferve flefh kept in it fweet, and even reftore it after it becomes putrid. It is therefore given with great fuccefs in putrid fevers, in the fea fcurvy, in dyfenteries, in mortifications, and in other diforders arifing from a putrid caufe, or attended with putrefaction, a draught of it being taken now-and-then, or even by way of common drink. But the ingenious

O genious

genious Mr. Bewly has invented a ftill
better method of exhibiting fixed air,
as a medicine : he directs a fcruple of
kali to be diffolved in a fufficient quantity (fuppofe a quarter of a pint, or
lefs) of water, which is to be impregnated with as much fixed air as it can
imbibe; this. is to be drunk for one
dofe *. If immediately after it a
fpoonful of lemon juice, mixed with
two or three fpoonfuls of water, and
fweetened with fugar, be drunk, the
fixed air will be extricated in the ftomach; and by this means a much
greater quantity of it may be given
than the fame quantity of water alone
can be made to imbibe. In this way
I have given it in the above diforders
with the beft effect.

But for the important difcovery of
the efficacy of this medicine in the
ftone and gravel we are indebted to

* Mr. Bewly directs it to be prepared in larger quantity
at a time, (as indeed it ought, in order to fave trouble)
and calls it his *Mephitic Julep*.

Mr.

Mr. Benj. Colborne. After long undergoing the fevereft tortures, unrelieved by other remedies, of which he tried all of any repute, he firft experienced its happy effects in his own perfon, and afterwards recommended it to many of his fellow-fufferers with the fame fuccefs. For a full account of its effects, with a variety of cafes, fee Dr. Falconer's Appendix to Dobfon's Commentary on Fixed Air, from which the following manner of preparing and ufing it is tranfcribed.

" Put two ounces and a half troy weight, or two ounces and three quarters avoirdupois, of dry falt of tartar into an open earthen veffel, and pour thereon five full quarts, wine meafure, of the fofteft water, that is clean and limpid, that can be procured, and ftir them well together with a clean piece of wood. After ftanding twenty-four hours, carefully decant, from any indiffoluble refiduum that may remain, as much as will fill the middle part of one of the glafs machines for impregnating water with fixible air. The alkaline liquor is then to be expofed to a ftream of air, according to the directions commonly given for impregnating water with that fluid. When the alkaline folution has remained in this fituation till the fixible air ceafes to rife, a frefh quantity of the fermenting materials fhould be put into the lower part of the machine, and the folution expofed to a fecond ftream of air, and this procefs repeated four times.

" When the alkaline liquor fhall have continued about forty-eight hours in this fituation, it will be fit for ufe, and fhould then be carefully drawn off into perfectly clean bottles (pints are, I think, preferable) and clofely corked up. The bottles fhould then be placed with their bottoms upwards in a cool place; and with thefe precautions it will keep feveral weeks,

3   and

and perhaps much longer, very good.

- - - - - - - -

" About eight ounces by meafure
have been taken thrice in twenty-four
hours, and have agreed well with the
appetite and general health; but I
apprehend moft people will think this
too large a quantity; and I believe,
that for moft cafes, two-thirds of a
pint of the alkaline liquor in twenty-
four hours may fuffice. Should the
bulk of the feparate dofes be thought
too large, the alkaline folution may be
made of double the ftrength; in which
cafe half the quantity will be enough.

" The times of taking three dofes
in the day, have been, I believe, pretty
early in the morning, about noon, and
about fix in the evening. If twice a
day, about noon and in the evening;
and if once, which in many cafes feems
fufficient for a preventative, about an
hour and a half before dinner. Common prudence dictates, that fuch a
remedy

remedy fhould be taken at fuch times as the ftomach is leaft likely to be loaded with victuals.

" I do not find, from obfervation or inquiry, that a rigid adherence to any particular regimen of diet is neceffary, farther than the ufual prudential cautions of moderation and temperance.

" The reverend Dr. Cooper has made ufe of fruit, wine, and other things fubject to acefcency, during the time of his taking the folution ; yet no perfon has received greater benefit. I however think it would be advifeable to abftain from acids, and from fuch things as are fubject to become acefcent, for fome time before, and alfo after the time of taking the dofes of the alkaline folution."

Mr. Bewly found his head affected by a dofe which he took, which alfo proved a pretty ftrong diuretic ; but it was a very large dofe, containing twenty-four ounces by meafure of

fixed

fixed air. In general it has no perceivable effects. If it fhould prove cold or flatulent to the ftomach, Dr. Falconer recommends a fmall portion of fpirit to be added. He fays too, that hot milk in the proportion of about one-fourth, is a very grateful addition, efpecially in cold weather, and tends much to reconcile it to the ftomach.

When the lungs are purulent, fixed air mixed with the air drawn into the lungs, has repeatedly been found to perform a cure.

The bark may be given with advantage in water impregnated with fixed air, as they both coincide in the fame intention.

Fixed air may be applied by means of a fyringe, or otherwife, to putrid ulcers, mortified parts, ulcerated fore throats, and in fimilar cafes, and it has been found to have remarkable efficacy. It may alfo be given internally at the fame time.

In

In putrid dyfenteries, and in putrid ftools, fixed air may be given by way of clyfter, as hath been obferved by the learned and ingenious Dr. Prieftley (whom I have the honour to call my friend) in the former part of this work. Fermenting cataplafms are of fervice chiefly as they fupply fixed air to the part.

In cafes of putridity, fixed air has been fuccefsfully applied to the furface of the body, expofed to ftreams of it. And there are other cafes in which it has been found ferviceable. Water impregnated with it is alfo an excellent cooling as well as ftrengthening beverage in hot relaxing weather, and it has befides the advantage of being pleafant to the tafte.

The virtues of water, impregnated with *hepatic air* may be collected from what was faid in the Introduction, concerning fulphureous waters.

F I N I S.